Qualitative Music Therapy Research

Qualitative Music Therapy Research

Beginning Dialogues

Edited By

Mechtild Langenberg
Kenneth Aigen
Jörg Frommer

Barcelona Publishers 1996

This book is published and distributed by

Barcelona Publishers
4 Whitebrook Road
Gilsum, NH 03448-0089

© *1996 Barcelona Publishers*

ISBN 0-9624080-4-2

Cover Illustration
by
Frank McShane

Contents

PART II: DIALOGUES

Acknowledgements

We would like to thank all the contributors to this book and all who helped to stay in contact over the long distances across the Atlantic Ocean. We are grateful to the Stichting Muziektherapie and the Fonds Muziektherapie van de Vereniging "BUMA" in The Netherlands, and the Foundation Gesellschaft der Freunde und Förderer der Heinrich-Heine-Universität Düsseldorf, Germany who sponsored the *First International Symposium for Qualitative Research in Music Therapy*. We would also like to thank Wolfgang Tress for his critiques and support of our efforts to develop qualitative research and for his help in developing the professionalization and theoretical foundation for the treatment method of music therapy detailed in Monologue 6. Special thanks are also due to Michael Langenbach who brought new and inspiring ideas into our group with his musical analyses resulting from his unique background as both a psychiatrist and musicologist, and for his help in translating many of the papers into English, our international communicative bridge.

Last but not least, we are very grateful to Kenneth Bruscia, a kind, sensitive and experienced music therapist and qualitative researcher who gave us the chance to publish the results of the Symposium in the form of this text. During the complex international communication process proceeding from the Symposium in 1994 and onward, through letters, faxes, telephone calls and his contributions in the text itself, Ken helped us to find ways through misunderstandings due to the presence of different social, cultural and research traditions in our group. He encouraged us to stay open minded, while providing space for a forum of discussion without any prejudices or intrusive corrections and criticisms of the authors.

Ken's support made possible the exploration of a wide range of opinions and an inspiring field of tensions. The Dialogues and Epilogue of this book are designed to provide an overview of these differences and tensions. Perhaps the candor of the authors and their willingness to engage in true dialogue can be an example for the type of process needed to develop clinical and research strategies which will advance the discipline of music therapy.

Mechtild Langenberg, Berlin
Kenneth Aigen, New York
Jörg Frommer, Düsseldorf
April 1996

Preface

Life is energy, rhythm and structure. Life is music. Music emanates from the wells of life. That is why music can heal and can damage. Energy streams of rhythm can be considerably disturbed by others.

This should be the starting point of a scientifically acceptable music therapy. A scientific music therapy should integrate its primarily episodic knowledge into the broad framework of medical treatments. Music is part of the most ancient and long-standing traditions of treatment. It is also part of the holistic art of healing and cannot do without this great tradition. It should not be considered a singular kind of treatment but a dimension in the process of healing. Music therapy should get into contact and into fine-tuning with other medical branches in order to develop its true potential for the benefit of patients. This will involve a difficult process of exchange and mutual respect with ample room for risks of misunderstanding. Those music therapists concerned about the scientific stance of their art will have to follow a rocky path in order to help ill and disturbed patients in the year 2000 and not to fall into the pitfalls of esoteric endeavor. These concerns will be important whether music therapy remains a treatment method incorporated into other models or if it yields an original and substantial contribution to the theory of disorders, their classification, nosology, diagnostics and differential indications. This remains an open question. However, it is only the maintenance of ideals and dreams which can further scientific knowledge.

I am extraordinarily pleased that the project embodied in this wonderful book, once itself just a dream, was successfully completed. Please excuse me for mentioning Mechtild Langenberg and Jörg Frommer in particular, both of whom prepared the ground for this Symposium in long and painstaking prepatory work. The scientific rigor of the Symposium was coupled with an attitude of friendly interrelating of all the discussants. I am sure that the authors in this book are willing to view their specialty of music therapy as a holistic contribution to health and to further an open discourse with the scientific traditions of the natural sciences and the humanities. I hope that this important book will find the international readership and warm acceptance it deserves.

Wolfgang Tress
Düsseldorf, Germany
April 1996

CONTRIBUTORS

Kenneth Aigen, DA, ACMT
Director of Research
Nordoff-Robbins Center for Music Therapy
New York University
New York, NY
USA

Dorit Amir, DA, ACMT
Department of Musicology
Bar-Ilan University
Ramat Gan, Israel

Jutta Baur-Morlok
Psychoanalyst
Düsseldorf, Germany

Kenneth Bruscia, PhD, CMT-BC
Professor of Music Therapy
Esther Boyer College of Music
Temple University
Philadelphia, Pennsylvania
USA

Jörg Frommer, MD
Professor of Psychosomatic Medicine
Otto-von-Guericke-University
Magdeburg, Germany

Carolyn Bereznak Kenny, PhD, CMT
Department of Music
Capilano College
Vancouver, British Columbia
Canada

Michael Langenbach, MD
Clinical Institute and Clinic for
Psychosomatic Medicine and Psychotherapy at
Heinrich-Heine-University
Düsseldorf, Germany

**Mechtild Langenberg, PhD, Diplom-Musiktherapeutin,
DGMT, DBVMT**
Professor of Music Therapy
University of Arts
Berlin, Germany

Gerhard Reister, MD
Clinical Institute and Clinic for
Psychosomatic Medicine and Psychotherapy at
Heinrich-Heine-University
Düsseldorf, Germany

Gerd Rieger, Diplompädagoge, Diplom-Musiktherapeut
Director of Absorption Center
Youth Community Center
Krefeld, Germany

Even Ruud, PhD
Professor of Musicology
Institute for Music and Theater
University of Oslo
Oslo, Norway

Henk Smeijsters, PhD
Co-Director of the Music Therapy Laboratory
Hogeschool Nijmegen
Nijmegen, The Netherlands

Andreas Stratkötter
Clinical Institute and Clinic for
Psychosomatic Medicine and Psychotherapy at
Heinrich-Heine-University
Düsseldorf, Germany

Wolfgang Tress, MD, PhD
Clinical Institute and Clinic for
Psychosomatic Medicine and Psychotherapy at
Heinrich-Heine-University
Düsseldorf, Germany

Prologue

Mechtild Langenberg

The *First International Symposium for Qualitative Research in Music Therapy* took place in Düsseldorf, Germany, in July 1994, at which time an international group of music therapy researchers began a formal collaboration. This community of researchers is just beginning to define itself and is entering into dialogue about research methodology, cultural identity and subjective influences on each researcher's approach. We are interested in developing qualitative research approaches to obtain a better understanding of our clinical work, our patients, and ourselves, while placing a high priority on communicating what we learn to other professionals. This book comprises an overview of the dialogue process of the group from 1994 to 1996.

Although the Monologues—six works describing different research approaches—provide an overview of different perspectives in qualitative music therapy research, we make no claim to have provided a complete survey.

In the Dialogues, ten responses are offered to the main themes which emerged from the discussions during the symposium. Many topics are examined upon which the various authors take opposing positions. These will provide fertile areas for future analysis and their resolution will encourage the development of standards among qualitative researchers in music therapy and related disciplines.

History of the International Symposium

There is a tradition in music therapy of bringing together individuals who have created training programs in international symposia and conferences. As pioneers, many qualitative researchers welcome opportunities to share their ideas and to contact others engaged in similar efforts to develop the discipline of music therapy through clinical work, research and training.

In 1978, Johannes Th. Eschen and Konrad Schily, together with the Gemeinnützige Gesellschaft für angewandte wissenschaftliche Forschungen mbH (GAW), organized the *International Symposium for Music Therapy Training* at the Gemeinschaftskrankenhaus Herdecke. In 1982, Barbara Hesser of New York University organized the *International Symposium on Music in the Life of Man: Toward a Theory of Music Therapy* at which working groups addressed questions in the areas of clinical practice, research, and training in music therapy.

Because of common interests, the qualitative researchers represented in this book have felt an increasing need to come together to create a forum to discuss their approaches and to create a supportive professional community. At times, this group will meet at larger conferences and sometimes we meet in smaller working groups where it is possible to go into more detail regarding issues in research methodology.

The results of research into music therapy are often difficult to present, at times reflecting the difficulty of the methodological problems involved in the research—this is part of the pioneer's work. Increasingly, music therapy is becoming more elaborated in the areas of clinical practice and research. There are post-graduate and doctoral programs at universities in many countries. We feel that it is important for music therapy researchers to meet in order to integrate their research programs in the academic sphere.

Musical works created during music therapy sessions have rarely been treated as objects of research, one reason why the academic discipline of music therapy has not yet been well established within the realm of professional psychotherapy. As a result, most music therapists who have professional training or university degrees are relegated to secondary positions and limited to auxiliary functions with the health professions. In these contexts, music therapy, with its nonverbal processes, often serves to prepare the patient for treatment or to enhance its effects. It is thus difficult to initiate research activities into the primary effects and uses of music therapy, or even to become integrated into research projects conducted by other professionals. There is then the additional challenge to maintain independence once the integration into the research programs of others has been achieved.

Interdisciplinary cooperation, however, is essential to take advantage of strategies which have already been developed in research on processes in psychotherapy. Yet, this poses the continual challenge to music therapy researchers of delineating music therapy as an autonomous research domain that can benefit from input from related fields. At Düsseldorf University, this cooperation was achieved by having a music therapist trained in music psychotherapy, a psychiatrist, and a psychoanalyst integrated into clinical work at the Department of Psychosomatic Medicine and Psychotherapy. Research in music therapy is integrated into the larger qualitative research program and has been developed in close connection to clinical practice and evaluation. With growing insight into the methodological complexity of our field, we have felt the need to exchange ideas on standards, values and guidelines in research.

Background of the Düsseldorf Project

In the department of Psychosomatic Medicine and Psychotherapy of the Heinrich-Heine University the importance of treatments such as body therapy, movement therapy, art therapy and music therapy has been acknowledged for quite some time. Patients at this facility suffer from a broad range of disorders such as psychosomatic disorders, neuroses and severe personality disorders. There is often a lack of self-awareness and sensitivity, an inability to differentiate emotions and feelings, and minimal contact with the inner and outer world. We try to integrate different treatment forms into a plan tailored to the unique needs of each individual. The inpatient and day hospital treatment units are unique models of integrated psychotherapy.

Music therapy, as one of the "specialized therapy forms," seems to be coming of age and developing into an independent and effective psychotherapy treatment. We use it in two ways: First, in addition to individual and group psychotherapy, every patient is assigned to a program of adaptive therapies such as social therapy, body therapy, art therapy or music therapy. Individual treatment plans are developed in team conferences.

Second, in a pilot project we use music psychotherapy as a primary therapy for selected patients when appropriate. This is possible because of the presence of a music therapist who has the position of a psychotherapist with academic training. The concept of the *Resonanzkörperfunktion* (resonator function) which I have written about elsewhere (see Monologue 6) is used in clinical and research work and provides the basis for our music therapy research project. This qualitative approach to evaluation dovetailed with existing interests at Heinrich-Heine University to support research strategies appropriate for examining psychotherapy processes. Jörg Frommer directs the Research Section for Qualitative

Methods in our department with which we have been cooperating since 1991.

Many researchers looking at verbal forms of psychotherapy have felt that the methodological instruments provided by nomothetical science are too unspecific to describe precisely what happens during therapeutic interactions. Prominent colleagues believe that distribution curves, formed on the basis of statistical group analyses, tend to cloud reality. They suggest a return to a more differentiated analysis of individual cases. One way of doing this is to try out various descriptive models and methods borrowed from the field of qualitative social research.

Qualitative social science traditionally deals with social conditions and specific subjective implications of individual behavior, taking into consideration idiographic and hermeneutic elements. Only through more careful examination of these various determinants do we find it justifiable to expect that we can grasp the course and outcome of psychotherapeutic processes in their complexity. This should lead to the ability to make general statements by comparing individual case analyses.

It remains to be discovered what exactly brings about a process of change in the interaction between patient and therapist and how to best describe these processes. The personal encounter in therapy requires research methods appropriate to the situation. These methods must be able to pick up different qualities of the work, in our case these are qualities of the encounter in the musical improvisation (see Monologue 6). These qualities include the exchange of thoughts, feelings and fantasies accompanying the encounter and, in particular, the qualities of the relationship formed by the personalities of patient and therapist. Research strategies have to be designed in the context of particular treatment methods. These are the guidelines along which music therapy in Düsseldorf is integrated into the research projects of the university department.

International Cooperation

We first developed the idea of an International Symposium for Qualitative Research in Music Therapy in 1990 when Wolfgang Tress became the head of the Department of Psychosomatic Medicine and Psychotherapy at the Heinrich-Heine University in Düsseldorf. He supported qualitative research approaches and initiated a Research Section for Qualitative

Methods.

In Germany, contact with David Aldridge of the Institute for Music Therapy at the University of Witten-Herdecke provided inspiration for our plans. We have engaged in discussions about research methodology since the early 1990s. Henk Smeijsters from the Netherlands, along with his international contacts, helped to prepare the symposium together with our co-sponsor, Stichting Muziektherapie. He has co-edited the *European Music Therapy Research Register* (Volumes I & II). International collaboration was broadened across the Atlantic when the present author presented parts of her work at the Conference of the American Association for Music Therapy (AAMT) in Cape Cod, Massachusetts in 1992. Discussions with Kenneth Aigen of the Nordoff-Robbins Center for Music Therapy at New York University showed that there were mutual interests with the New York group. At New York University, Barbara Hesser has developed a doctoral program that has trained experienced clinicians in qualitative research methods since 1986. Two of her students, Dorit Amir from Bar-Ilan university in Israel and Kenneth Aigen, are participants in the symposium group of researchers. I, Mechtild Langenberg, have been the head of the Department of Music Therapy of the University of the Arts in Berlin since 1995. Cooperation continues with a proliferating working group of students, postgraduate candidates and interested colleagues.

PART I: MONOLOGUES

MONOLOGUE 1

The Role of Values in Qualitative Music Therapy Research

Kenneth Aigen

THE VALUE-BOUNDEDNESS OF INQUIRY

As I prepared this work I found it particularly difficult to decide how to begin. Any discussion of values is bound to arouse passions, particularly when addressing a diverse audience such as the worldwide community of music therapy researchers. After all, consciously or unconsciously, we build our identities and live our lives according to our core values. Discussing values challenges us to examine our own beliefs and, by extension, our selves, to determine how well our lives reflect those things which we believe to be most important. As well, the presence of shared values is what holds communities together and the examination of values can be felt as a threat to the group with which we identify.

At first, being aware of these considerations led me to think that it might be helpful to distinguish between (1) exploring the role of values in research from (2) specific values that any researchers (including myself) might hold, and to limit my remarks to the first of these topics. In this way, I hoped to establish a common ground for discussion without having to argue for or evaluate the utility of specific values. However, in actual practice this distinction became difficult, if not impossible, to maintain. I soon realized that acknowledging the necessity of exploring the appropriate role of values in research *is itself a value judgment*—performing the exploration in (1) is actually an example of (2).

Thus, my starting point for this discussion is that it is contradictory and potentially disingenuous to have a "values-neutral" discussion of the role of values in research. My decision to choose this topic stems from certain beliefs and preferences. These beliefs affect the way that I frame and discuss this issue and they have a rhetorical or persuasive character. Here are a few assumptions that I would like to offer which guide my discussion:

1) A value-free science is neither possible nor desirable.

2) Anything I say about research relates to *all* of our activities as researchers, including our interactions and relationships with the following individuals: research participants; students who may be researchers in training; conference and symposia attendees; and, fellow researchers. These are not merely observations for others or for later on when involved in research projects, but instead are guidelines and criteria that should be applied to this Monologue itself. Our professional values should be *reflexive*, simultaneously applicable to the domain we are studying, our activities while conducting research, and the verbal and written forums in which we communicate with fellow researchers and present our findings. The beliefs that guide our interactions in daily life should also apply to our relationships with each other as members of a research community and to the participants in our research.

3) Qualitative research—taken in the broad sense of the term to include many non-positivistic approaches to inquiry—is based upon unique values which suggest specific ethical guidelines. Moreover, different approaches to qualitative research incorporate and emphasize different values. Thus, it is the researcher's responsibility and obligation to articulate these within the context of the research report.

4) These values can play a role in developing indigenous standards for evaluating qualitative research in music therapy.

Because it can bear different interpretations, it may be helpful for me to elaborate on how I am using the term "values." I have in mind the social sense of the term which refers to "the ideals and customs of a society toward which the people of the group have an affective regard. These values may be positive, as cleanliness, freedom, education, or negative, as cruelty, crime, or blasphemy" (Random House Dictionary, 1973).

Although values may have a moral basis they do not necessarily have to, thus allowing for the presence of other considerations such as aesthetic ones. For example, because of an aesthetic preference scientists may place a value on parsimony or elegance in choosing among competing theories although there may be no moral reason for this preference. In this way, we can see that a group's values reflect their preferences and are not necessarily identical with a code of ethics, for example, something with which values can be mistakenly identified. Of course, in one culture the aesthetic choice may have an underlying ethical component and in another it may not. This makes it difficult to establish understandings of values across cultures.

In spite of the inherent difficulties in its discussion, I have two primary reasons for believing that this topic is an essential one for music therapy researchers to consider. First, I subscribe to a philosophy of science which recognizes that practitioners in a given domain share certain values, experiences, beliefs, and forms of knowledge, both tacit and explicit. By bringing these elements into our forms of professional discourse we can more fully articulate our communal identity and develop research protocols and standards consonant with our core beliefs. Our knowledge base will then have an internally consistent, although certainly not infallible, foundation.

Second, I also believe that the role of values is one of the characteristics which differentiates the more progressive qualitative approaches (such as *Phenomenology, Hermeneutics, Naturalistic Inquiry*, and *Heuristic Research*) from the more traditional qualitative approaches (such as *Transcendental Realism* and *Grounded Theory*) and from quantitative research. The fact that there is a need for a book such as this one suggests that some of us feel that what we do under the label "Qualitative Research" is fundamentally different from traditional research and does not merely reflect the utilization of alternative data sources or types of analysis. My sense is that this difference lies in the recognition that what we call "knowledge" is less objective and immutable than it is personal and context dependent. Therefore, to fully understand a research study, for example, it is necessary to understand the personal context in which the research study is embedded.

THE RESEARCHER'S PERSONAL CONTEXT

Traditional accounts of science hold that the intrusion of values contaminates research—hence, there is no reason to know anything about the researcher to understand the research. The relevant background for establishing the meaning or significance of a study is the professional context, which often consists of related, previous studies and existing theory—these connections are typically established through literature review sections. Yet, in addition to placing a study within a theoretical tradition I believe that there is an additional subtext to the literature review. The researcher is also engaged in establishing competency in the eyes of the reader by referring to the "correct" or "important" previous studies and forging a common ground with the reader by establishing a shared professional history.

When we recognize a researcher's references we are reassured that we share a common training, history, and destiny, and a whole host of tacit assumptions are activated. These assumptions allow us to read the work and experience its meaning by drawing upon a common experiential base. Conversely, when we do not recognize a researcher's references we experience the work as that of a "foreigner," someone from an alien culture with whom we may not share a sense of history, and by extension, a common experience to draw upon. Thus, although it would probably be denied by traditional researchers, the review of the literature section of any research document serves to establish a common ground of values in which the exchange of ideas can take place.

Qualitative researchers actively embrace this important function through providing the *personal context* in which the work is embedded as well as the professional one. Instead of establishing the necessary connections to readers in an oblique or unconscious way, we recognize the importance of directly and overtly accessing our readers' body of assumptions and common experiences in order to make the full meaning of the research document available to them. Any work depends upon context for its meaning. Qualitative researchers have an expansive view of what comprises the relevant context and acknowledge that highlighting the personal context is important in allowing all facets of a research document to be revealed.

In the various qualitative research approaches, different labels are used and different uses for this information are emphasized. In Hermeneutic research one offers a *Self-Hermeneutic*, in Phenomenology this is called an *Epoché*, in Naturalistic Inquiry we refer to the *Stance of the Research-er*, and Heuristic Inquiry can include movement between the personal and the public throughout the research document.

While the content is influenced by the focus, scope, and particular research method, there are a number of common elements across these different methods. Although not an exhaustive list, some of these aspects of the researcher's value system include: 1) the researcher's motivation for conducting the study, in personal and professional terms; 2) prior experiences and beliefs which have shaped the area of inquiry and which influence data-gathering and analysis; 3) the researcher's group member-ships—such as gender, ethnicity, socio-economic status, position of employment—which are offered so that the political and social forces that may have been active in the study can be considered openly; 4) the nature of the relationship between the investigator and the research participants, whether this latter group consists of a professional panel, clients in therapy or their family members, or other interviewees; and, 5) ways in which the researcher was changed by the process of research.

The purpose behind providing this information is three-fold, simulta-neously serving methodological, ethical, and presentational ends. The methodological dimension itself has two aspects: The first is to provide sufficient information about the researcher's preconceptions and influences in order for readers to be able to account for the effects of these in the final product as well as to gain a more comprehensive understanding of the research findings. Second, the process of engaging in this self-reflection helps the researcher to be as forthcoming as possible about these influences in order to minimize their unconscious effects.

In terms of ethics, it is essential for researchers to disclose any information that bears on their having a vested interest in obtaining certain research results, such as is the case when clinician-researchers study their own work.

In terms of presentation, this information is engaging as well as useful to readers. Establishing the researcher as a human being with particular values, concerns, fears, interests, and insights, assists the reader in becoming more involved in the topic and findings of a given study. There is a large personal and professional risk in revealing our selves in this way and it is important for us to support each other by recognizing the ethical and methodological advantages of doing so.

Knowing the reasons behind a given study helps the reader to identify with the researcher and, by extension, with the researcher's interests. Through revealing this type of personal information the researcher creates a vicarious experience in the reader, allowing the reader to connect to an analogous experience in his or her own history. The result is that the reader is better able to apply the results of the inquiry because they will now have personal meaning as well as be of professional interest.

As an example, I would like to offer my own work as the Director of Research at the Nordoff-Robbins Center for Music Therapy at New York University. Here, I am often in the position of studying and evaluating the work of colleagues, including peers and supervisors. These are important facts to be aware of for any consumer of my research who would be justified in wondering whether or not this position has unduly compromised my research. Yet, it is also important to discuss how this level of access has helped my research in specific ways.

In the work discussed later in this monologue, *Here We Are in Music: One Year with an Adolescent, Creative Music Therapy Group*, I studied a music therapy group led by two co-workers with whom I shared an office. The obvious danger here was that I would look at their work less critically because of a reluctance to damage either our professional relationship or personal friendship. On the other hand, my prior relationship to them, and the ongoing access that I maintained, allowed me to forge long-term, trusting relationships in which they could speak with greater candor and provide me with deeper insight into their clinical work. Thus, it is more correct to say that my personal context influenced my work and made it possible than it is to say that it biased my work or rendered it excessively subjective. The challenge for any researcher is to examine the personal context, gain insight into its interaction with the field of study, and include these considerations in the research report so that the reader can judge if they were handled responsibly.

As human beings, our everyday notion of "understanding" goes beyond that which is typically considered to be appropriately scholarly, academic, or detached. "Understanding" has emotional, intuitive, and value-laden aspects that connect to the basic existential concern of making sense out of our experience and our existence. In psychological terms, I would say that affect and cognition are related to a degree that we tend not to acknowledge in research activities. By providing this personal, human context as part of our research, we are bringing the potential for a deeper degree of understanding to ourselves and to our readers.

SELF STUDY: COMBINING CLINICAL
AND RESEARCH ROLES

Whenever we study clinical work—either our own or that of others—specific issues arise which impinge on the research process. At an early stage of the study mentioned above, I found myself combatting feelings of boredom while observing the group. I disagreed with the structured approach being implemented and found my thoughts occupied by what I would do differently rather than being focused on what the group members were actually experiencing. In other words, my differences as a clinician were obscuring my ability to function as an observant researcher. Fortunately, the research approach I subscribe to—Naturalistic Inquiry—encourages the researcher to maintain an ongoing investigation of his or her emotional process. Through the mechanisms of my research *support group* (Ely et al., 1991) and *reflexive journal* (Lincoln & Guba, 1985) I was able to discover and explore the source of these feelings in order to not project them onto the research participants, thus minimizing their distorting effect on my research.

One point that I would like to draw from this is that whether we study our own clinical work or that of others, there will be unique issues to contend with, opportunities for insight, and precautions that must be taken. Neither situation is inherently more ethical or more methodologically advantageous than the other.

These considerations bring us to a central issue: What are the ethical and methodological concerns when a researcher is studying his or her own clinical work? Many of us are motivated to do research precisely because we want to find out more about clinical practice, often our own. We should acknowledge that there are serious obstacles to consider when we examine how to do this in a way that is clinically responsible and methodologically sound. On the other hand, as a qualitative researcher I believe that method should be subordinated to, and derived from, the content of that which we would like to study. Therefore, I prefer to develop procedures and relationships to address these difficulties, rather than abandon the idea of combining the roles of clinician and researcher.

The important thing to keep in mind is that there are both potential advantages as well as disadvantages to a client in participating in a course of therapy which is being (or will subsequently be) researched. As well, there are advantages and potential difficulties to the researcher in combining these roles. Our position as researchers should be to anticipate, find ways to manage, and discuss in our reports, the potential difficulties, and to make the most of the potential benefits. In so doing, we will protect the interests of our clients, avoid contaminating our research, and attract the attention of clinicians who otherwise may be skeptical about our research results.

First let us look at why it might be unethical to research one's own work. From a methodological perspective, one possibility is that our analyses as researchers will suffer because we are interested in seeing particular outcomes which will support the value of our work as therapists. Thus, our research interpretations run the risk of not being credible. In terms of clinical ethics, it is possible that these needs will lead us—either deliberately or unconsciously—to influence the client in a way that will lessen the benefits of the therapy. Here, our clinical choices will be affected by our research agenda and the client's needs become secondary. Related to this is that a client changes or unconsciously colludes with the therapist in order to be a "good" subject for research.

In a sense, these issues are not specific to research as they also can come into play in the non-researched clinical situation. Therapists have certain expectations of clients and clients can have their actions affected by what they perceive as therapist expectations. These are issues which clinicians are expected to deal with in supervision. The difference in research is that one must consider the dynamics of the *research relationship* in addition to those of the therapeutic relationship. This type of examination can—and should—be conducted through the mechanisms that I mentioned previously, the support group and reflexive log.

Something which is by definition particular to research is that the therapist's interventions are changed by the research: either we become more active or interventive in order to make sure that "something happens" or we become more inhibited because of a reluctance to have our work looked at under the microscope of research. There is also a danger that we become less patient or accepting of clients if the client's growth process does not fit the timetable of our research project.

Because of these considerations, some may believe that it is actually unethical to research a course of therapy while it is in progress. It could be argued that research, of necessity, changes the therapy and that the changes are necessarily negative for the client regardless of the precautions taken. Therefore, any research on clinical work should take place only once the client has finished treatment.

I disagree with this position for three reasons: First, the potential conflicts or drawbacks for the clients can be responsibly managed through the appropriate procedures. Second, if we know that, once concluded, a course of therapy will subsequently be researched then the same potential problem areas are activated; merely waiting to engage in research activities until after the therapy has concluded does not mean that the dynamics of the research relationship will not come into play while the treatment is proceeding. Third, I believe that there are also *benefits* to clients of having their therapy researched which can, at times, outweigh the potential problems.

It is presumed that a course of therapy that is researched will undergo more scrutiny, will be looked at in more detail and from more perspectives than would a non-researched course of therapy. The client should benefit from this increased level of attention as the treating therapist gains more insight into the client's process. Also, some clients may benefit from the feelings of importance or by feeling that they have something to contribute by participating in research projects. Last, whether or not a client is actively involved in the research—such as is the case with a procedure called *member checking* (Lincoln & Guba, 1985)—the client is nonetheless contributing to a certain construction or interpretation of the clinical music therapy experience. In this way, the client can have direct impact on the profession and on the way that future services are delivered. The perspective to keep in mind is that clients are one of the primary stakeholders in any research project and their participation in research studies gives them a voice where otherwise they may have none.

Researching therapy—particularly one's own work—changes the process. This in and of itself is not a criticism. The researcher's obligation is to be cognizant of these changes and discuss how they influenced the music therapy process. We will then be able to know to what extent the findings of a researched course of therapy are applicable to non-researched therapy processes.

In the United States, much of the impetus behind the interest in qualitative research is due to the lack of relevance of traditional research to clinical concerns. I see this issue of applicability not just in methodological terms but in ethical terms. Because music therapy is a service profession, and because most music therapists will never have the resources or expertise to engage in systematic research, I believe that those of us with these resources have an obligation to develop studies which clinical music therapists find interesting, which relate to their work, and which will, directly or indirectly, help them in their work with clients.

The notion of relevance is perhaps the most basic premise from which our research should proceed. This is why we must sanction, and find ways to support, the concept of the clinician-as-researcher. Experienced clinicians working on an advanced level are in the best position to know what research topics will be applicable to their work. Using their expertise, either as participants or leaders of research projects, will help ensure that the products of our research are read and applied by those in the best position to make use of them.

DISCUSSION OF *HERE WE ARE IN MUSIC*

Moving from the general to the specific, I would like to discuss some aspects of the study *Here We Are in Music* (Aigen, in press) from the perspective of what my own values were and how they influenced the course of the study and the presentation of its findings. Briefly, this study details the course of music therapy over a one-year period for a group of developmentally-delayed adolescents at the Nordoff-Robbins Center for Music Therapy at New York University. The group members, ranging in age from thirteen to seventeen, all had significant communication problems and exhibited a variety of autistic tendencies. I videotaped all of the sessions from a small booth adjacent to the therapy room and my data consisted of these tapes, my own notes made directly after the sessions and after viewing the tapes, and interviews with the two therapists.

What I call my value system is more appropriately considered a context dependent process, a type of engagement, than a formal and static set of rules that is universally applied. Different situations affect me in a different ways, stimulate different thoughts, values, and ethical considerations, and demand individualized responses from me as a researcher. Here are some of the considerations that were most prominent for me during this study:

1) The research should have relevance for the therapists in the study and, in some way, help them to better understand and help their clients.

2) It was important to include information from the multiple perspectives represented by the variety of individuals involved in the study, the four clients, two therapists, and myself as the researcher. Conveying the sense of what it was like to be a member of this group was especially important.

3) The narrative form I chose for reporting the findings had to reflect the content of what I wanted to convey rather than merely the procedures I followed. The form is integral to the content and the two should be consistent and mutually reinforcing.

4) Understanding processes in music therapy requires contextualizing them in terms of the particular individuals participating in the research. Much as in the contextualization of the research product, fully understanding these processes required getting a feel for the research participants as individuals.

I believed these four concerns to be consistent with one another—a strategy developed to meet one often addressed another as well. For example, in the study there are many instances of detailed descriptions of sessions. I saw this description as an important part of my research focus because the nature of group music therapy process with developmentally-delayed adolescents is not something that has been written about extensively. This extensive description served two of the above considerations. By providing these detailed accounts of life in the therapy group the nature of the experience for its members could begin to be apprehended by the reader, thus addressing my concern for including multiple perspectives. This detail is also of use to other music therapists in determining the study's applicability. By knowing what actually happened during a substantial portion of the sessions, these therapists can ascertain the degree of similarity between their own clients and clinical work, and those in the study. In the qualitative approach, it is this determination—rather than constructing a representative sample, for example—that determines the generalizability of findings.

After a brief introduction, the study itself begins with four *constructs* (Ely et al., 1991), monologues written from the perspective of the research participants, in this case the four clients. These constructs can consist of either direct quotes or thoughts, feelings, and statements which the researcher believes are typical of the participant. I included these constructs primarily because I wanted the reader to have a sense of the clients as people and to be able to ground the interpretive material in terms of specific individuals, not just in the class of "developmentally-delayed adolescents." This also functioned to bring the group members' perspectives to the report, albeit in a limited fashion. I felt that it was important for the group members' voices to speak directly to the reader—this was *their* story. Because their disabilities rendered them unable to meaningfully participate in an interview, I felt that the construct was the best alternative.

In an effort to secure multiple perspectives, I interviewed both therapists on two occasions. In these sessions, I asked them about their rationale for different interventions, what they thought the group dynamics were and how these were affecting the different group members, and, what their experience was like in the group. Interestingly, there was an important peripheral benefit from these sessions. Both therapists reported that the extensive interviews stimulated them to think about the group in different ways and to gain insights into their own roles which they might not have otherwise considered. Here is an example where the research activity—rather than the finished project—brought unintended benefits to the clients by helping the therapists to be more aware of their own implicit clinical strategies and the patterns that emerged in the group process.

This was one way in which my presence as a researcher directly affected the domain of the study. I have found that qualitative research is necessarily an interactive process where the process of doing research has a profound effect on the product. Therefore, discussing factors which influence the research process belong in the research product. We are always studying ourselves regardless of whatever else we are studying. This is why I recommend discussing the parallel process of self-exploration concomitant to the exploration of our research domain. The experiences we have as researchers change us as people which in turn impacts significantly on the research. As participant researchers, we exert change forces on the field of study as the field simultaneously changes us. Therefore, we are always *part of* the study, inseparable from it, regardless of whether our overt focus is outward—such as in this study—or inward—such as in a study like Kenneth Bruscia's (1995) *Modes of Consciousness*. Discussing ways in which we were affected by our research will invariably add richness and deeper levels of understanding to our work.

Another way in which this mutual interaction can be seen in *Here We Are in Music* is through looking at the creation of data through filming the therapy sessions. In a very basic sense, by undertaking the filming of the group I created the clinical record which was used by the therapists each week in reviewing the session. For those unfamiliar with the details of the Nordoff-Robbins approach, each session is videotaped and the therapists review the tape, creating detailed written indexes of the session. The therapists' impressions of the value of the session is strongly mediated by its taped legacy. As the filmer, I decided where to focus the camera and how to frame each shot, moment-by-moment. The resultant portrait of the session was created by the considerations I felt to be important.

Hence, my research agenda strongly influenced the therapists' perception of the therapy which in turn strongly influenced their clinical strategies and the therapeutic process which I was observing. There is a circular aspect to this generation of knowledge which would violate every canon of science which portrays the researcher as the neutral, undisturbing observer. Not only was I disturbing what I was observing but in a sense I was helping to create it!

Yet this is not so problematic when we realize that all scientists create their data, not in the sense of fabricating it but in the sense of selecting what is important. A fact or observation only becomes a piece of data when it exists in relation to a given theory or research focus. Researchers in all domains choose their theories or focus—these are not handed down in an a priori manner. In this sense, there is an interactional element between all investigators and the domain they are investigating, of the same type, but maybe not to the same degree, that occurred in my study. Again, to a return to an oft-repeated theme: It is the researcher's obligation to set forth the considerations going into the selection process rather than to avoid selection or deny that it takes place. To engage in research is to engage in selection, to make choices. To engage in research as a participant-observer is to interact with and have an effect upon the domain that one wishes to study. What we should focus on as researchers are mechanisms to take advantage of this interaction to the benefit of research participants and our studies.

In the final write-up of this study, I informed the reader of these considerations regarding my filming as well as the aspects of my biography which affected my selection process. These included my own clinical preference for working improvisationally and with an awareness of group process. Thus, when I report as an important finding that these group members exhibited the classic stages of group process as discussed by authors such as Irwin Yalom (1985) and benefitted from the therapists working with an understanding of group process, the reader knows that I have a predisposition to see things in this light. It then falls to the reader to determine if my preconceptions unreasonably distorted my representation of the nature of the group experience, or if my conclusions are warranted by the detailed description of sessions and multi-layered presentation that I also provide as a way of judging the interpretations.

One might be tempted to go one step further and say that it is possible that as the researcher I can stack the evidence by selecting only those incidents for report that support my interpretations. I would answer—somewhat surprisingly to some—that this is exactly what I do. I build my interpretations from the data that have an impact on me where the degree of this impact is not solely determined by frequency of occurrence. To do this would be to use a misplaced *quant*itative criterion. This does not meant that I ignore data but that I endeavor to make my interpretations account for all of the data that my judgements and expertise deem to be important. The checks on this process are the procedures involved in my data analysis to establish the trustworthiness of my report.

As a qualitative researcher I understand that a research report has a rhetorical function: This is to convince the reader that what I experienced as important is, in fact, important and that the knowledge I gained from the study is worth accessing and applying for oneself. This does not mean that I believe that research is propaganda. It does mean that all writing forms and narrative structures affect us in overt and unconscious ways to influence how we judge a given document. In traditional research writing, the subjective "I" is eliminated; the resulting reports sound more authoritative because the absence of the first person endows statements with the prestige and "objectivity" of that which is universal as opposed to that which has its source in a specific individual. The point is that eliminating the subjective "I" is just as much a deliberate strategy to sway a reader's thinking as is utilizing the subjective writing voice.

Part of my agenda in writing the report for *Here We Are in Music* was for the reader to gain a vicarious experience—I wanted to bring the reader as close as I could to the emotional and musical experiences which characterized the sessions. I was not merely content to convey information through my writing, instead wanting to engage the reader on a variety of emotional, musical, and intellectual levels. The vehicles I chose for this included the constructs as described above; detailed accounts of volatile, emotionally charged therapy sessions; and, musical transcriptions of improvised songs.

My reasons for this were varied: On one level, I saw myself as an advocate for the clients in the group. I wanted their essential humanity to come through so that whoever came into contact with this work would see new potentials in clients similar to those in the study. I also felt that there were lessons to be drawn from the study that I did not see but that others might. By engaging readers through their own vicarious experience, I hoped that the study itself could be maintained as a living document that readers interact with rather than simply read and absorb in a passive manner. Last, I wanted this work to get inside the reader, activating his or her own professional history and values. I feel that it is through helping readers to internalize our written work—by relating it to their own lives and professional experiences—that we as researchers can have the most beneficial impact on music therapy. As we develop this fledgling area of qualitative research in music therapy, we should be more willing to adapt and experiment with those presentational forms that will best facilitate the application of our work.

DEVELOPING STANDARDS FOR EVALUATING QUALITATIVE STUDIES

Because qualitative approaches are becoming more commonly applied to music therapy it is important to develop standards for evaluating qualitative music therapy studies. This means evaluating both the process of research as well as the product of research, the final report. Although this is an important distinction to make, in this preliminary work I will not distinguish between evaluating findings and evaluating the actual conduct of research.

My belief is that conventional scientific criteria are inappropriate devices for assessing qualitative studies. Yvonna S. Lincoln and Egon G. Guba (1985) offer the concepts of credibility, transferability, dependability, and confirmability as the qualitative analogues to the traditional criteria of internal validity, external validity, reliability, and objectivity. Without going into any of their arguments I will just repeat their basic rationale for this. Stemming from the observation that traditional inquiry has a different epistemological basis from that of qualitative inquiry they simply say that "different basic beliefs lead to different knowledge claims and different criteria" (p. 294).

In the balance of this Monologue, I will discuss some of the considerations that should have a prominent role as we begin developing or choosing criteria appropriate for evaluating qualitative studies.

In the qualitative approach, such criteria have a different function from what we are accustomed to in human science research. In psychology, for example, a study must meet the standards listed above, otherwise it is considered to be seriously flawed and not worth considering. In contrast, I do not think that the standards we develop should function in the same way as a "litmus test" in determining the value of a given report. They offer guidelines for evaluation and no single one nor combination is either necessary or sufficient for an evaluative judgement to be made. I say this because, in the qualitative approach, method is neither a guarantor nor an arbiter of truth. Because so much of qualitative research is dependent upon the skills, personal qualities, and insight of the researcher, it is possible that a given method could be meticulously followed and still not produce valuable or trustworthy findings. Similarly, a researcher might not use any of the mechanisms suggested but still produce a worthwhile study. These criteria, then, are best considered tools that should help us to better understand why some studies are interesting and useful and why others seem to be of limited value. In no way should they be considered rules which must be followed. In this chapter, I have tried to focus on those standards tied to specific values. For a comprehensive approach to the question of generating trustworthy findings and evaluating them, I again recommend the work of Lincoln and Guba.

Considerations from Music Therapy as a Service Profession

I would like to begin with a consideration from my earlier illustration regarding the identity of music therapy as a service profession—our discipline exists to help individuals in a temporary or prolonged state of intensified need through music. Hence, any research project should facilitate this general mission. Of course, this can be drawn in very broad terms so that our definition of "help" is an expansive one, to include things such as: immediate, tangible benefits to the participants in a study; generating information demonstrated *by clinicians* to be of use to them in their activity as clinicians; empowering marginalized classes of clients through giving them a voice in the professional literature; exciting and inspiring clinicians who are always in danger of professional burnout; and, obtaining more societal resources for those who make use of music therapy services. This is only a partial list to provide a sense of the multiple ways in which the criterion of "helping" can be construed.

The important point is that somewhere, somehow, we as researchers must be held accountable for the uses, or lack thereof, to which our research products are put. In the United States, music therapy research has never been held in high regard by the majority of practicing clinicians. By seeing relevance or application as an ethical as well as a methodological concern, qualitative researchers can take a progressive stand in remediating one of the long-standing problems with music therapy research. To do this, in our work as doctoral advisers, members of journal editorial boards, coordinators of scientific programs at conferences, and most importantly, as researchers, we must hold up our own work and that of our colleagues and students to a simple standard when we review an article, dissertation, or conference proposal: Who has been or will be helped by this work? This should be our first question in evaluating any piece of research.

The Notion of Value

When we evaluate research we are seeking to establish its value. I would like to examine two separate aspects of this notion of value: One is *accuracy* or what is often referred to as validity, truth, or credibility. The other component is its *usefulness* by which I mean its potential for application, relevance, interestingness, or the degree to which its content is compelling for its intended audience. Accuracy is not to be considered in terms of precision but instead as *appropriate representation*. For example, a metaphor can be quite appropriate in capturing a mood yet still be impressionistic rather than specific, and poetic truth can be accurate without being precise.

Traditionally, there has been a trade-off between accuracy and usefulness, especially when accuracy is conceived of in quantitative terms as precision. One is then forced to choose between the two—an increase in accuracy can mean a decrease in usefulness. A music therapist who uses a measure such as duration of eye contact for determining the efficacy of treatment is falling into this trap.

There are two lessons that I would like to draw from this. First, we must not equate value with accuracy. In ascertaining the value of our research we must include its potential usefulness as being of at least equal importance. Second, usefulness and accuracy need to be seen as related rather than opposed. Let me briefly expand on this point.

I have been using a somewhat awkward construction in this discussion: the term "interestingness." My intent is to suggest that when clinicians find a piece of research to be interesting or even compelling, this in and of itself has a bearing on both aspects of value. The fact that it is found interesting has obvious bearing on the "usefulness" component as its interest is derived from the way that it reflects clinical concerns held by practitioners. Its connection to the "accuracy" side is not so obvious however. What I am suggesting is that when clinicians find a research work interesting, one reason they may do so is because the work faithfully reconstructs important aspects of their experiences as clinicians. A false or inaccurate reconstruction would not be responded to in the same way. Taken in this way, we can see that one possible arbiter of the faithfulness of our research reports to the domain they are purporting to represent can be the response of those clinicians who have lived through similar experiences; in a general sense, their interest can bear on the authenticity of the way the clinical reality is reconstructed through the research product.

Multiple Perspectives

Another concept which has potential to serve as a criterion for evaluating qualitative studies is the use of *multiple perspectives*. This is important for a few reasons: First, is the idea that the realities studied by researchers are just that: multiple in character rather than singular. The use of multiple sources of data in method is thus consistent with the epistemology underlying many forms of qualitative research.

Also important is the recognition that researchers are not in an epistemologically superior position to that of research participants. The perspectives of participants are equally important to those of researchers.

Another reason for the use of multiple perspectives is the fallibility of the human instrument known as the researcher. Because qualitative researchers often rely on their own intellectual capacities rather than on formalized tests or inventories in data analysis, there is the potential to allow personal frames of reference to unnecessarily limit research findings. The use of multiple perspectives can serve to take advantage of our human analytic capacities while minimizing the possibility of developing incomplete or distorted portraits.

The final consideration here is that knowledge itself is a multi-leveled phenomenon—methods which draw upon a variety of types of knowing will necessarily be more complete than those restricted to that which can be expressed in propositional form, for example.

In sum, the use of multiple perspectives has methodological and ethical rationales: It is consistent with ideal of equality between researcher and participant to which many qualitative researchers aspire; it provides participants with a voice in research; it creates a more complete document; and, it can serve as a check on the limitations of the researcher as the human instrument. Yet, it would be a mistake to assume that the idea of using a panel is to reduce potential subjectivity by seeking a consensus to arrive at the one "true" description. The purpose of utilizing multiple perspectives is to generate multiple descriptions or constructions and to examine each as valuable in its own right. The idea is not to combine them or to determine that the objective truth lies in the area in which the multiple descriptions overlap or have common elements.

There are many ways in which multiple perspectives can be integrated into a study. Carolyn Kenny (1987) and Mechtild Langenberg et al. (1993) are among those who have created research panels in order to provide for fuller and more complete portraits of the processes that they studied. For Carolyn Kenny, the panel served to provide feedback from a variety of professional viewpoints on her theoretical construction; for Mechtild Langenberg the panel provided data used in evaluating the utility of her theoretical construction of the "resonator function."

I have alluded to the concept of the support group in describing one of the ways in which I maintained the integrity of the research process during my study. This group of peers serves the researcher much as a supervision group serves the therapist. Here, the multiple perspectives served to widen my perspective as a researcher and to help me avoid unconscious bias in my data collection. Many qualitative researchers write about the depth of personal involvement maintained in their research, including things such as: the passion they feel about their research; how research is an interactive process which, when performed well, has a transformative impact on the researcher; and, the intense frustrations and joys characteristic of engaging in qualitative studies. They also note how valuable it is to have a group of individuals who can perform the varied functions of offering support and encouragement at difficult stages of the research process as well as challenging the researcher's interpretative process. An important value that qualitative researchers share is a sense of being part of a research community bound by a particular attitude to life, one which recognizes our intuitive, symbolic, and affective processes—as well as our intellectual ones—as vehicles for obtaining insight. The use of the support group extends this value by creating a vision of colleagueship where emotional support exists together with intellectual rigor and challenges.

In his study, *Modes of Consciousness,* Kenneth Bruscia (1995) uses the concept of multiple perspectives in an interesting way. Before detailing this I would like to offer some background. At New York University I teach a doctoral seminar in which each student offers a critical presentation of a qualitative music therapy research study which the entire class has read. One of the most common criticisms of existing studies has been that the researcher made inadequate use of the various potential multiple perspectives. Thus, the research document appears to be excessively self-contained.

In this class, the study that was evaluated most favorably was, in fact, *Modes of Consciousness* in spite of the fact that it did not make use of any of the possible multiple perspectives delineated thus far. There was no research panel, support group, or set of multiple participants in the study. What there was, however, was a multi-layered use of four levels of experience, which the author notes as being roughly analogous to Jung's four functions: sensing, feeling, thinking, and intuiting. The need for a multi-layered presentation was met in this study not through the use of multiple participants but through examining the rich layers of experience utilized by an advanced clinician as he goes about his work. Ken Bruscia's method of analysis and presentation created a holistic portrait of being a GIM (Guided Imagery and Music) guide in a way that proved to be insightful and satisfying.

Considerations from Our Identity as Musicians

The last issue that I would like to discuss in this regard is vitally important but probably the one around which it is most difficult to speak. This relates to our identity as musicians and the values that flow from this aspect of our group membership. What values do we inherit from being part of the worldwide family of musicians? What role do we want these values to play in our research? And, how are we to ascertain the integral implementation of these values? These are they types of questions that I have in mind.

Primarily, we have an obligation to music itself and to the musical experience. Much of the impetus behind the interest in qualitative research is due to the fact that quantitative research does not handle the phenomenon of music very well. Clinicians look at quantitative reports and find nothing in them that reflects the musical aspects of their clinical experience. Because qualitative research does not place the same types of constraints on what constitutes legitimate data sources, we have available the nature of the musical experience as an area for research. This exploration was an important part of Dorit Amir's (1992) study on *Meaningful Moments* discussed in Monologue 5 of the present text.

There are many ways to bring music into our research reports and activities. One concrete way is to include musical examples through the use of written transcriptions, audio tapes and video tapes. In *Here We Are in Music* I felt that it was essential to include musical transcriptions because important components of the group members' experiences were *contained in* the music. To know what the group members lived through requires knowing the music which embodied and expressed their individual struggles and collective process.

Another important strategy is to make music and the musical experience the actual focus of our research. This is probably the most important area for us to be looking at and the one that many of us—myself included—seem to shy away from. Certainly the two studies by Langenberg, Frommer, & Tress (1993; 1995) represent some of the few good examples in this area as does the phenomenological study by Forinash & Gonzalez (1989).

If as qualitative researchers we are committed to generating holistic understandings of music therapy process, this necessitates finding ways to include in our research the musical experiences essential to our clinical practice. The degree to which our research efforts meet this holistic injunction necessitating the inclusion of music appears to me as one of many possible criteria along which to evaluate our research efforts.

As musicians we are first and foremost *listeners*. We know how to listen *through* sound to hear the underlying "story" behind the tones, rhythms, and silences that comprise music. As music therapists we learn how to hear not only the archetypal elements of the piece, and not only the elements that reveal our personal stories to us, but also to hear the story of another soul expressed in music. We learn to enter the inner reality of another human being through his or her music. What is it to say that music reveals a person's inner psychodynamics if not that the narrative that comprises the individual's personal history and journey of self-understanding and development is thereby conveyed?

Thus, it would seem important for us to recognize this value of learning to hear story through music and finding ways to bring this into our research efforts. Again, there are many possible ways of doing this. One is to use story as a narrative structure in our research reports. These stories can comprise clinical vignettes relevant to understanding the clients with whom we work and the role of music therapy in their lives. Or, they can be more metaphoric in character. Similarly, we can allow the telling of stories stimulated by music to be one way of collecting data. Here, I think of the way in which the research panel in the Langenberg et al. articles were encouraged to share their imagery and to expand upon these images to include elements of narrative. The unfolding of imagery typical of GIM practice also reflects a recognition of the importance of story, seen in the study by Kenneth Bruscia referred to above.

As a species we have always taught, learned, and communicated the nature of our existence through story. Our encounter with music in the clinical setting creates its own family of stories. We should understand the story form as an important cognitive vehicle for the transfer of knowledge, especially for those forms of knowledge which unfold in time and require an aesthetic or symbolic form to begin with, such as music.

Although solo performance certainly exists as an important phenomenon, music is essentially a communal experience. More often than not, music is created in groups of at least two, such as in individual music therapy when client and therapist play together. Creating music involves the simultaneous fitting together of a multitude of individual voices. Musicians must share their aesthetic space in a way that is more demanding than in any other art form.

As we learn how to fit our individual needs and voices into the communal expression we learn to respect the value of the individual in relation to the group. Each individual and each voice performs a different function which contributes to the whole in a unique way. Playing as a group means hearing each individual's contribution and making room for it in the communal creation. There is a democratic, pluralistic ethic that seems integral to our identities as musicians.

This ethic should also play a role in all of our research activities, including presentations and other interactions with colleagues. Compared to other health care professions with more recognition and prestige, music therapy has been a marginalized profession. One characteristic of groups who feel that they have been discriminated against is to adopt the trappings and dynamics of the group or groups in power. (See a fascinating article by David Read Johnson, 1994.) To me, this explains why music therapists have traditionally courted favor with medical professionals and often adopted a medical model of research and treatment.

Yet it is possible for us to avoid this trap and instead maintain our identities as musicians, thus creating a new vision of a health care profession. Certainly we can draw upon our roots as musicians to hold on to the more pluralistic aspects which recognize and respect the value of the individual.

The egalitarian values which spring from this musical self-identity can also be applied to our relationships with research participants. Rather than treating them as passive, inert "subjects," we can build a model where research is looked at as a collaborative venture between research-er, therapist, and client, with each having input into all aspects of the research cycle: formulation of topic; implementation; analysis; and, reporting of findings. For example, Heron (1981) discusses a research approach in which participants contribute "to the creative thinking that generates, manages, and draws conclusions from, the research" (p. 153). For those of us who subscribe to a clinical value system broadly described as humanistic, these procedures will help to build a research approach consistent with these principles. They will also help to ensure the ethical use of participants and the relevance of research findings.

As I said previously, these recommendations are suggested guidelines, none of which is either individually or collectively necessary for a given work to be considered a bona fide piece of research. I believe that judging the value of research should be done flexibly and based upon the merits of the individual project rather than mechanically according to adherence to a pre-determined set of procedures. Adherence to method is no substitute for experience, insight, intuition, and good judgement. These uniquely human capacities used by clinicians and by researchers in their professional activities should ultimately be the same ones used in our evaluation of research. To extend Guba & Lincoln's point about developing paradigm specific standards for evaluation, perhaps we should examine the knowledge claims made in individual studies and apply those evaluative standards appropriate to the specific claims.

Because of the importance placed on research by service institutions, private and public funding bodies, and medical authorities, as researchers we have unique opportunities to define music therapy and serve as emissaries to the outside world. Along with this opportunity is a responsibility to define and represent the profession in a way that honors the experiences of clinicians and clients and that is true to our ancestral roots as artists and healers.

REFERENCES

Aigen, K. (in press). *Here we are in music: One year with an adolescent, creative music therapy group.* Nordoff-Robbins Music Therapy Monograph Series #2.

Amir, D. (1992). *Awakening and expanding the self: Meaningful moments in the music therapy process as experienced and described by music therapists and music therapy clients.* Doctoral Dissertation, New York University. UMI Order # 9237730.

Bruscia, K. E. (1995). Modes of consciousness in guided imagery and music (GIM): A therapist's experience of the guiding process. In C.B. Kenny, (Ed.), *Listening, playing, creating: Essays on the power of sound.* Albany: State University of New York Press.

Ely, M. with Anzul M., Friedman T., Garner, D., and Steinmetz, A.M. (1991). *Doing qualitative research: Circles within circles.* London: The Falmer Press.

Forinash, M. & Gonzalez, D. (1989). A phenomenological perspective of music therapy. *Music Therapy*, *8*(1), 35-46.

Johnson, D.R. (1994). Shame dynamics among creative arts therapists. *The Arts in Psychotherapy*, *21*(3), 173-178.

Kenny, C. B. (1987). *The field of play: A theoretical study of music therapy process*. Doctoral Dissertation, The Fielding Institute. UMI order #8802367.

Heron, J. (1981). Experiential research methodology. In P. Reason & J. Rowan, (Eds.), *Human Inquiry: A Sourcebook of new paradigm research*. New York: John Wiley.

Langenberg, M., Frommer, J. & Tress, W. (1993). A qualitative research approach to analytical music therapy. *Music Therapy*, *12*(1), 59-84.

Langenberg, M., Frommer, J. & Tress, W. (1995). From isolation to bonding: A music therapy case study of a patient with chronic migraines. *The Arts in Psychotherapy*, *22*, 87-101.

Lincoln, Y. & Guba, E. (1985). *Naturalistic inquiry*. Newbury Park, California: Sage Publications.

Yalom, I. (1985). *The theory and practice of group psychotherapy*. New York: Basic Books.

Because their work is so integral to the ideas expressed in this paper, I have provide the following additional works of Guba & Lincoln, although they are not specifically cited.

Guba, E. & Lincoln, Y. (1981). *Effective evaluation: Improving the usefulness of evaluation results through responsive and naturalistic approaches*. San Francisco: Jossey-Bass.

Lincoln, Y. & Guba, E. (1990). Judging the quality of case study reports. *Qualitative Studies in Education*, *3*(1), 53-59.

Qualitative Single-Case Research in Practice: A Necessary, Reliable, and Valid Alternative for Music Therapy Research

Henk Smeijsters

INTRODUCTION

During the past few years at the Music Therapy Laboratory in Nijmegen, a qualitative research method has been developed for use in practice in music therapy with individual clients (Smeijsters, 1991; Van den Hurk & Smeijsters, 1991; Smeijsters & Van den Hurk, 1993a, 1993b, 1994; Smeijsters & Van den Berk, 1994). Despite the fact that the use of experimental quantitative outcome research is often justified for social and political reasons—the underlying idea being that this is a way for music therapy to prove its usefulness to policy makers—in psychotherapy research this model is being increasingly questioned.

The fact that criticism is being voiced must not become an excuse to allow the move away from the natural science model to end up in methodological quicksand. Qualitative research is not easier than quantitative research, it is different from it. Adhering to the accepted criteria for sound scientific research requires some adaptation but the criteria themselves must not be tampered with.

This work discusses the necessity for doing qualitative single-case research.

QUALITATIVE SINGLE-CASE RESEARCH VERSUS QUANTITATIVE GROUP EXPERIMENTS

In quantitative research, the use of calculating devices results in two steps of abstraction from everyday experience which produce numerical representations of this experience. A felt experience like being sad can be put into words as a first level of abstraction. If it is put into figures, e.g., 1-10, a second level of abstraction takes place.

Quantitative research starts with a theory and existing concepts about reality. From this theory, hypotheses are inferred in a deductive way. The hypotheses are tested in an experimental setting to discover effects of treatment. Client groups are selected by sampling and treatment variables are carefully selected and kept stable in time. Effects are assessed by calculating group means and significance.

In qualitative research the approach is very different. Qualitative research refers to a method aimed at describing and conceptualizing processes occurring in a natural therapeutic setting uninfluenced by experimental manipulations (Bogdan & Biklen, 1982). Only the first level of abstraction is used in verbal descriptions of experience. So descriptions where sounds rather than words are used to describe experience—as in music therapy—are even closer to experience because sounds can be analogies for direct experience (Smeijsters, 1993).

Qualitative research is inductive and lends itself to generating hypotheses. Concepts develop while observing processes in a natural situation. The procedure of formulating concepts is based on openness to, and feedback from, the data.

In qualitative research, data typically consist of experiential information from the study participants. In single-case designs, the object of study is an individual client or an existing group. There are no samples, as such, but rather examples. Because the focus is on personal processes, intrasubject developments are more important than within or between group means.

Shortcomings of the Quantitative Group Experiment in Measuring Effects

Qualitative single-case research has enjoyed considerable attention within the field of psychotherapy research in recent years (Cook & Campbell, 1979; Kiesler, 1983; Strupp, 1990; Hilliard, 1993). Current methods of effect measurement in groups have come under criticism. They are of little value when studying the process of change in psychotherapy. In the "black box" model of behaviorism, scores on pre- and post-test administrations of psychological tests are compared; the development that takes place between pre-test and post-test is not considered (Greenberg, 1986). During treatment, small changes take place and the study of these changes offers insight about when and how effects occur and what triggers them.

The experimental group approach in psychotherapy research is also criticized for the heterogeneity of the clients within and across both the experimental and control groups. Focussing on changes implies looking at the individual because all changes are individual and mean changes do not exist. Mean changes are artifacts.

Other objections include ethical and internal validity problems with regard to the control group, and the complexity of the therapeutic situation and the limited possibility and desirability of isolating, manipulating and stabilizing independent variables (Greenberg, 1986; Kazdin, 1986). Another criticism is that while measuring instruments allow for collection of data that can be directly compared among researchers, they always reduce reality to operationalized variables thus excluding other data from constructions of reality. A limited number of isolated variables simplifies the complexity of the natural situation (Hutjes & Van Buuren, 1992). Combined quantitative and qualitative research with measuring instruments and clinical observations by music therapists shows that there is a discrepancy between what can be measured by measuring instruments and what is freely observed by music therapists (Meschede, Bender & Pfeiffer, 1983).

In recent years single-case research has come to be conceived as a legitimate alternative. Hilliard (1993) defines single-case research as intrasubject research which focuses on the individual's internal changes over time. Generalization is not based on the averages of representative samples, rather it is achieved by replicating individual cases. In Hilliard's opinion, the single-case design can be either experimental or observational; the data processing can be quantitative or qualitative. The approach can be either one of testing hypotheses or of generating hypotheses. Thus, single-case research is not equivalent with qualitative research.

In music therapy treatment, isolating variables and subjecting the client to an experimental procedure is not always feasible or desirable. It is also important for the music therapy process to be able to develop freely (Aigen, 1993). Hence, single-case research should be observational and non-experimental. Moreover, due to the fact that measuring instruments are insufficiently reliable and valid as yet (Aldridge, 1993), and because standardized instruments only reflect part of the experiences in music therapy, single-case research should be qualitative. Since there is a lack of theory from which hypotheses can be drawn, it should be generating hypotheses (Remmert, 1992).

To summarize, the best approach for music therapy research at present is an observational, qualitative, hypotheses-generating, single-case approach.

The methods of treatment that are developed can be hypotheses that may be subjected to experimental testing and possibly quantitative, single-case research at a later stage.

While numerous traditional case studies of music therapy have been carried out, the amount of qualitative single-case studies and ideas about this kind of research has been steadily increasing in recent years (Forinash & Gonzalez, 1989; Kenny, 1989; Amir, 1990, 1992; Tüpker, 1990; Langenberg, Frommer & Tress, 1992, 1993, 1995; Aigen, 1993, 1996; Aldridge, 1993, 1994; Bruscia, 1993, 1995; Van den Hurk & Smeijsters, 1991; Smeijsters & Van den Hurk, 1993a, 1993b, 1994; Smeijsters & Van den Berk, 1994).

THE NON-SCIENTIFIC CASE STUDY

One way of studying individual cases in natural situations is the traditional case study. This type of study however is generally not afforded much scientific status because it fails to meet the requirements considered important for research (Kazdin, 1986). It is unclear, for example, how much of what is reported in a case study as being the therapeutic process is the result of conscious or unconscious subjective selection on the part of the therapist. What data will be selected at another moment or by another person? The selection of data can result in an unjustified suggestion of a link between treatment and effect and increases the likelihood of overlooking alternative explanations. A case study of this type provides the reader with insufficient information to be able to check the accuracy of the conclusions. It is also uncertain whether the coding of the selected data fits the reality being described. This is equally relevant for both treatment and its effect. Because of all the various possible distortions caused by selection, uncontrolled coding and arbitrary argumentation about treatment and effect, this type of case study has to be labelled unscientific.

Using the concepts of reliability and validity, we can take a more detailed look at the above-mentioned problems (Campbell & Stanley, 1966; Yin, 1989; Hutjes & Van Buren, 1992). These concepts are used in quantitative research, too. Some qualitative researchers use different concepts such as credibility, applicability, consistency, and neutrality to stress the differences between quantitative and qualitative research (Lincoln & Guba, 1985). However, it seems as if these new concepts are closely linked to the old ones. In qualitative research the old concepts still can be used if their contents become accommodated to the characteristics of qualitative research.

Research is reliable as long as the selection of material is neither arbitrary nor dependent on coincidence. For instance, when an audiotape or videotape of a music therapy session is watched by only one observer who carries out a single observation without a measuring instrument the resulting data depend on the chance selection that the observer happens to make at that one moment. As these data are determined by chance they are non-reliable. Conclusions based on this selection have no scientific significance.

Construct validity refers to the accurate representation of events by the constructs (codes) used to describe them. This leads to a common problem in music therapy whenever musical processes are described using terminology derived from psychotherapy. The same musical event may be described differently by music therapists according to their preferred theoretical model. This in itself is not necessarily contradictory because a situation can be viewed from various perspectives. If the same detail is given entirely different labels, however, its construct validity becomes dubious.

Internal validity refers to whether the effect can be shown to be a consequence of the method used. Was the client cured by the treatment or by other factors? In a traditional research design using an experimental and a control group, the potential influence of factors such as simultaneous events, maturation, spontaneous recovery, statistical regression, the influence of repeated measurement, etc. (see Campbell & Stanley, 1966) is accounted for because it can be assessed by looking at the control group. Because the case study has no control group the multiple variables which might produce an effect are not checked. The therapist often merely describes what happens during therapy and concludes that if an effect occurs it is caused by the treatment that preceded it. Almost no consideration is given to competing variables and alternative explanations.

Without a representative sample drawn from a given population, the external validity of a case study—its applicability to other situations—is low. This is compensated by the fact that because the natural setting in which the case study occurs is not subject to experimental manipulations, its similarity to actual clinical practice is greater than is that of the controlled experiment.

THE SCIENTIFIC CASE STUDY

Central to what follows is a conception of the qualitative, non-experimental scientific case study which does not rely on statistical tests and in which treatment is not manipulated. How can its reliability and validity then be ensured?

Reliability

A separate point highlighted by, among others, Bogdan and Biklen (1982), is worthy of special attention because it often features explicitly in the argument used by music therapists and music therapy researchers. It is the view that qualitative research is concerned with subjective meaning rather than objective truth.

It has often been suggested that the essence of music therapy is lost in the process of quantitative research. This essence is identified as the personal experience of the client and the music therapist during music therapy including images and feelings (Hesser, 1982; Forinash & Gonzalez, 1989; Osborne, 1989; Amir, 1990; Tüpker, 1990; Aigen, 1993; Forinash, 1993). In these examples, the researcher can have various roles: Researcher and music therapist can be the same person (Forinash & Gonzalez), the researcher can act as a participating observer alongside the music therapist (Amir) or the researcher can adopt a role distinct from the subjects (Osborne).

The personal feelings, sensations, images and ideas of the client and the music therapist must be part of research. Just as in treatment, in research the empathic countertransference of the music therapist provides information useful in understanding the experiences of the client. It can be argued that research can only address essential aspects of music therapy treatment via the subjective experience of the music therapist during treatment.

If it is stated that this should be the only rationale for doing research, it raises new questions. First: does the essence of music therapy consist only of the experiences of the client and the music therapist or are there other aspects—such as process and musical events—that need to be addressed? (see Bruscia, 1993)

Second: a strong emphasis on the music therapist's experience seems open to question because these experiences can change in time within the individual and between individuals. When it is agreed that experiential meaning instead of truth is the essence of research, doing research means "re-searching" this experiential meaning. This does not mean looking for truth, because personal experiences of people always are true and cannot be false, but it does mean that more personal experiences—from the same and separate individuals—can throw light upon it. These other experiences do not conflict with the experience of the music therapist but instead enrich it. If only the music therapist should be allowed to be the researcher, then, in a paradoxical way, one supposes that only the music therapist possesses the truth.

The view that objectivity obstructs subjectivity without which the essential music therapy process cannot be understood (Tüpker, 1990), seems not to take into account that subjectivity can have two distinct meanings. On one hand, it can merely refer to one's private experience; on the other, it can be equated with the idiosyncratic, or that which depends on the selection of meaning by one person at one particular moment in time. The music therapist, while reflecting the experience, selects out of this experience "meaningful moments" (Amir, 1992).

When a process involving a client is subjected to an experience oriented observation carried out by someone else, it is important that this observation comprises more than just one observer's personal experience at any one moment in time. Some form of repeated or intersubjective experiencing is essential from the point of view of research.

Trying to eliminate the idiosyncratic refers to the rationale of reliability. What possibilities are there to fulfill this rationale?

Tüpker (1990) proposed a controlled subjectivity which entails the music therapist being trained in the detection of countertransference. In many countries, educated and credentialed music therapists are trained in searching for countertransference. This training is a necessary but not a sufficient precondition for doing research and guaranteeing reliability. Reliability resembling the test-retest reliability of traditional research can be increased when the music therapist as a researcher repeats the same observation at different times. It is not possible to repeat the treatment, but it is possible to listen to the audiovisual recordings, read the reports and go into the experience again.

Interrater reliability can be increased by involving several independent observers. Observing means experiencing feelings, images and sensations. The first step would be to split the roles of music therapist and researcher. Repeated observations by the music therapist, by an independent researcher and by other observers can be used during the treatment process.

After a research project has been completed, repetition is possible by employing a detailed research report which allows a second independent researcher to mentally reconstruct the chain of evidence at some later date (Yin, 1989; Hutjes & Van Buuren, 1992). Recording the chain of evidence in a report can be compared to the job of a detective who has to precisely record the data on which conclusions are based. The detective not only looks for the selection made out of the data (reliability), but also inquires into the way the selected data were coded (construct validity) and the way the coded data were connected by the first researcher (internal validity). In this way, the research can be replicated by analyzing it on paper.

This method involves at least making four types of reports: the research proposal which includes the research methodology to be followed; the raw data (recordings, reports, interviews); the analyzed data reflecting the researcher's selections, generalizations, and interpretations; and, the finished written product. Because an article gives only a condensed representation of the course of research and does not offer an opportunity to consider alternatives, the rough data and analyzed database belonging to the research must be made accessible within ethical bounds.

Construct Validity

If in research a hypothesis is used as starting point, it is essential to define the constructs in the hypothesis precisely. For example, what is the meaning of the phrase, "The client is relaxed"? How is this relaxed state manifested and how is the degree of relaxation measured? To address questions such as these, Hutjes & Van Buuren (1992) use the terms "inventory" (the phenomena that constitute the construct) and "operations" (the way a phenomenon is registered).

If, as in qualitative research, existing constructs are not used as a starting point and the constructs are allowed to emerge from the data, several different sources need to be utilized. This principle is known in research literature as triangulation. It entails the use of several independent observers, various techniques of collecting data (such as observation, or interviews), or the use of diverse theoretical models.

Several observers are asked how they would describe the phenomenon. Various data collecting techniques give different kinds of information and diverse theoretical models offer several theoretical constructs that help to code the phenomenon. It is possible to ask how constructs are related and which constructs fit best.

In grounded theory (Glaser & Strauss, 1967; Strauss & Corbin, 1990) constructs are deliberately left open when answering the question "What is happening here?". The description and the naming of phenomena are constantly adapted until they fit the event as well as possible. After the first selection of constructs has taken place the function of the construct is that of a sensitizing concept which directs the process of searching. In this research method there is continual verification and falsification.

For example, if in the initial stages of diagnosis certain factors seem to point towards a compulsive personality (Van den Hurk & Smeijsters, 1991), this construct becomes a hypothesis and the material is inspected in order to find evidence for or against it. In this case a construct only remains useful if symptoms such as skepticism and a strong need for order and intellectualization (Cullberg, 1988) are detected both in musical and non-musical behaviors.

The construct validity is strengthened by describing and naming the musical processes as intersubjectively as possible and subsequently linking them to existing psychopathological or psychotherapeutic constructs (Maso, 1989). This requires careful consideration of whether a link to existing constructs is possible at all. The musical process and the existing psychopathological or psychotherapeutic constructs should fit together as well as possible. Here too, verification and falsification by related constructs must be conducted continually.

Another way of looking at triangulation is not as a dialectical process of verification and falsification but as a process of accumulating non-conflicting pieces of information. As is the case with reliability one source cannot falsify another, but two sources can provide a more complete description than one. This procedure, which also improves reliability, allows phenomena to be highlighted in a variety of ways and therefore to be labeled differently.

Internal Validity

The least a therapist can do in establishing internal validity is to register events which take place concurrent with therapy, e.g., changes in the situation at home, other treatment, weather conditions, hobbies, relationships. However, there are also several specific methodological measures which can be taken in order to check for internal validity.

Pattern matching or structural corroboration (Guba & Lincoln, 1981; Yin, 1989) refers to the procedure whereby preceding treatment a prediction is made that a particular pattern will occur if treatment is effective, the alternative being that a different pattern will occur if treatment has no effect. This method corresponds closely to the formulation of outcome goals according to precise operational definitions. The music therapist determines beforehand what changes will occur in the client's music if treatment is effective.

For example, if the client is unable to introduce any kind of form into the music, the therapist predicts that by improvising on polarities (such as hot-cold) the client will eventually spontaneously improvise within an A-B or A-B-A form. It is also possible to represent the idea as follows: When the client is able to play an A-B form, there must be an observable independent variable which in this case would be the thematic improvisation on polarities.

A second example links music therapy to non-musical behavior. In the treatment of the client with compulsive personality disorder, it was inferred that clinical goals like not being upset when locked up in an elevator, deciding spontaneously to go with a car to a garage, leaving for holidays without an endless list of precautions, and changing relationships, were effected by the free musical improvisations. This was made possible because of analogues between experimenting in musical improvisations and behavior outside music therapy (Van den Hurk & Smeijsters, 1991; Smeijsters, 1993; Smeijsters & Van den Hurk, 1994).

If the predicted pattern does not occur with the relevant treatment, if it occurs with a different treatment or without the relevant treatment having taken place, it must be concluded that there is no causal link between treatment and effect.

A method similar to pattern matching is time-series analysis in which the assumption is made that an effect is preceded by a particular sequence of treatment phases. For example, in the case of compulsive personality disorder, the process of working through grief in music therapy started with the exploration of musical elements which made possible the musical expression of feelings. In a subsequent case (Smeijsters & Van den Berk, 1994) the hypothesis that concentrating on musical processes precedes loosening of hidden feelings was affirmed.

When a particular effect is indeed preceded by a sequence of phases: A must precede B, B must not precede A; A must always be followed by B; and, B can only occur after a certain period. (Yin, 1989)

These techniques are not the only ones to guarantee internal validity. Other techniques that can be used during research are: "disciplined subjectivity" (Erickson, 1973; Tüpker, 1990), "peer debriefing" and "member check" (Guba & Lincoln, 1982; Hutjes & Van Buuren, 1992). In disciplined subjectivity, researchers reflect critically on their own interpretations. Peer debriefing means that the researchers ask colleagues whether they agree with their interpretations. In member checking, the client is asked if (s)he agrees with the interpretations. During treatment this can be a problem because it influences treatment. It can be used immediately after a treatment phase has finished.

A client with musicogenic epilepsy (Smeijsters & Van den Berk, 1994) often corrected the interpretations of the music therapist and the researcher. She questioned the hypotheses that movement could guard against epileptic fits, that fits were evoked by associations and that she was able to influence the fit at the beginning.

Advocates of qualitative research often argue that replication is impossible because every client and every moment is unique. Despite the fact that, phenomenologically speaking, every client, therapist, intervention, and moment indeed is unique and therefore impossible to replicate (Giorgi, 1985; Tüpker, 1990; Aldridge, 1993), this view is too dismissive of the similarities among clients, therapists and interventions. Therefore, the use of multiple-case studies (Miles & Huberman, 1984; Hutjes & van Buuren, 1992) is highly recommended whenever practical. To follow Bruscia (1993), qualitative analysis can be aimed at discovering aspects of phenomena unique and common to various cases.

Replication means replicating within an ongoing case or between different cases. In a reversal design, after an initial baseline period in which no treatment is given, treatment and baseline periods are regularly alternated. The idea is that when effects correspond with the alternation of the presence of music therapy, the cause cannot be attributed to any other external variable, provided no other independent variable alternates simultaneously.

In reversal designs, treatment is withheld which raises serious ethical problems. These problems can be avoided when there are normal holidays which can serve as a baseline. Another problem with this design arises when, after treatment, a carry over effect occurs and the value of the dependent variable does not fluctuate. If the treatment really has a lasting effect then it is not possible to see it fluctuate with the presence and withholding of treatment. Here, internal validity is not guaranteed.

The multiple baseline design makes use of parallel behaviors, parallel situations or parallel cases. While treating different behaviors of one client, the same behavior of one client in different situations, or the same behavior of several clients, treatments start at different times after a baseline period. If changes only occur after treatment it is likely that the effect is being caused by the treatment. After all, another variable which by chance coincides with the beginning of the treatments and which is causing the effect, would have to be constantly occurring at exactly the same time as the different treatments start.

A problem of this design—when one is aiming at influencing different behaviors of one person or a given behavior of one person in different situations—is the assumption that one behavior does not influence another and that there is no carry over from one situation to another. The client appears merely as a sum of discreet behaviors and situations. This is in conflict with the idea of a personal gestalt. When using several clients this problem does not exist.

In multiple-case studies, replication is literal when the treatment is repeated in the same way in a new case. A theoretical replication involves altering variables in the repeated study and predicting that the effects will change, too (Yin, 1989). A theoretical replication also can take uniqueness into account.

Last, but not least, replication can be fulfilled after research has finished by a second researcher who re-searches the chain of evidence.

External Validity

Case study research is not based on a representative sample of the population. Essentially, the results are only valid for that one case. However, a single case can represent other similar cases. It is then known as a typical case (Hutjes & Van Buuren, 1992). In a multiple-case study the individual cases can be manipulated to a greater or lesser degree in order to discover whether similar cases show similar patterns and differing cases different patterns (Hutjes & Van Buuren, 1992).

For example: a music therapy method for treating depression which has been developed on the basis of case study research must be applicable to each new depressive client and must lead to similar results.

CONCLUSION

As far as research is concerned music therapy is in an awkward position. Now that the inadequacies of quantitative experimental group research models are becoming apparent within the world of established psychotherapy research, music therapy researchers are also more willing to turn their attention to qualitative single-case research. Because the scientific tradition within music therapy is still relatively young, music therapy is in danger of both skipping stages in its scientific development as well as reverting to outdated positions.

With regard to the danger of skipping stages it should be acknowledged that quantitative research is a real option and that sometimes it is appropriate. As far as the other danger is concerned it is incorrect to assume that new paradigm research is completely new. In fact it can hardly be called a new paradigm at all, because for years the phenomenological method dominated European psychology. It was superseded by experimental and statistical methods because these methods seemed to comply better with criteria that were considered important. This meant that a methodological approach which was found to be relatively robust was declared universally applicable. As a consequence, in many cases the object of study was rendered subordinate to the method.

However, movements such as humanistic psychology began to emphasize human experience and the accepted methodology was questioned once again. Human experience is not standard, average or isolated. The same goes for the therapeutic process.

A struggle seems to have erupted between quantitative and qualitative researchers at present. But is this really an either/or situation? Are the two really comparable? A quantitative method can answer different questions from a qualitative one. Quantitative and qualitative methods should be incorporated into music therapy research in such a way that the chosen method of research depends on the question and the object—or subject—to be studied rather than the other way around. A research method is a means not an end.

In this article, it was argued that choosing a qualitative single-case method does not relieve one of the obligation to comply with scientific criteria. Questions such as the following are fundamental to scientific research: Has the phenomenon been represented as completely as possible? Has the phenomenon been adequately conceptualized? Is enough known about factors influencing the phenomenon? And, in what respects is the phenomenon similar to other phenomena and in what respects different? Factors such as reliability, construct validity, internal and external validity are all issues qualitative researchers must take into account.

The need for either a quantitative or qualitative research method depends on the nature of the question to be researched. Because single-case research is an intra-subject research method it yields insight into changes the individual client undergoes during the process of music therapy. The term "qualitative" refers to an openness to events, the development of concepts in ongoing interaction with reality, and the generation of hypotheses. This Monologue offers a methodological framework for qualitative single-case music therapy research. It first describes the weaknesses of the traditional case study and subsequently suggests techniques designed to ensure the reliability, construct validity, and internal and external validity of qualitative single-case research.

REFERENCES

Aigen, K. (1993). The music therapist as qualitative researcher. *Music Therapy*, *12*, 16-39.

Aigen, K. (1996). The role of values in qualitative music therapy research. In M. Langenberg, K. Aigen, & J. Frommer (Eds.), *Qualitative research in music therapy: Beginning dialogues.* Phoenixville, PA: Barcelona Publishers.

Aigen, K. (in press). *Here we are in music: One year with an adolescent creative music therapy group.* Nordoff-Robbins Music Therapy Monograph Series #2.

Aldridge, D. (1993). Music therapy research II: Research methods suitable for music therapy. *The Arts in Psychotherapy, 20,* 117-131.

Aldridge, D. (1994). Single case research designs for the creative arts therapist. *The Arts in Psychotherapy, 21*(5), 333-343.

Amir, D. (1990). A song is born: Discovering meaning in improvised songs through a phenomenological analysis of two music therapy sessions with a traumatic spinal-cord injured young adult. *Music Therapy, 9*(1), 62-81.

Amir, D. (1992). *Awakening and expanding the self: Meaningful moments in the music therapy process as experienced and described by music therapists and music therapy clients.* Doctoral Dissertation, New York University. UMI Order # 9237730.

Bogdan, R. & Biklen, S.K. (1982). *Qualitative research for education: An introduction to theory and method.* Boston: Allyn and Bacon.

Bruscia, K. E. (1993). A framework for qualitative research in music therapy. Paper presented at the *VII Congress of Music Therapy,* Vitoria, Spain.

Bruscia, K. E. (1995). Modes of consciousness in Guided Imagery and Music (GIM): A therapist's experience of the guiding process. In C.B. Kenny (Ed)., *Listening, playing, creating: essays on the power of sound.* Albany, NY: State University of New York Press.

Campbell, D.T. & Stanley, J.C. (1966). *Experimental and quasi-experimental designs for research.* Chicago: Rand McNally.

Cook, T.D. & Campbell, D.T. (1979). *Quasi-experimentation: Design and analysis issues for field settings.* Boston: Houghton Mifflin.

Cullberg, J. (1988). *Moderne psychiatrie.* Baarn: Ambo.

Erickson, F. (1973). What makes school ethnography ethnographic. *Anthropology and Education Quarterly, 4*, 10-19.

Ferrara, L. (1984). Phenomenology as a tool for musical analysis. *The Musical Quarterly, 70* (3), 355-373.

Forinash, M. (1993). An exploration into qualitative research in music therapy. *The Arts in Psychotherapy, 20*, 69-73.

Forinash, M. & Gonzalez, D. (1989). A phenomenological perspective of music therapy. *Music Therapy, 8*(1), 35-46.

Gembris, H. (1991). Musiktherapie und Musikpsychologie. *Musiktherapeutische Umschau, 12*, 279-297.

Giorgi, A. (Ed). (1985). *Phenomenology and psychological research.* Pittsburg, PA: Duquesne University Press.

Glaser, B.G. & Strauss, A.L. (1967). *The discovery of grounded theory.* Chicago: Aldine.

Greenberg, L.S. (1986). Research strategies. In L.S. Greenberg & W.M. Pinsof (Eds.), *The psychotherapeutic process. A research hand book.* New York: The Guilford Press.

Guba, E. & Lincoln, Y. (1981). *Effective evaluation: Improving the usefulness of evaluation results through responsive and naturalistic approaches.* San Francisco, CA: Jossey-Bass.

Guba, E. & Lincoln, Y. (1982). Epistemological and methodological bases of naturalistic inquiries. *Educational Communication and Technology Journal, 30*, 233-252.

Hesser, B. (1982). Research position paper. Presented at the *International Symposium on Music in the Life of Man.* New York University.

Hilliard, R.B. (1993). Single-case methodology in psychotherapy process and outcome research. *Journal of Consulting and Clinical Psychology, 61*(3), 373-380.

Hurk, J. van den & Smeijsters, H. (1991). Musical improvisation in the treatment of a man with obsessive compulsive personality disorder. In K.E. Bruscia (Ed.), *Case studies in music therapy.* Phoenixville, PA: Barcelona Publishers.

Hutjes, J.M. & van Buuren, J.A. (1992). *De gevalsstudie.* Meppel: Boom.

Kazdin, A.E. (1986). The evaluation of psychotherapy: Research design and methodology. In S.L. Garfield & A.E. Bergin (Eds.), *Handbook of psychotherapy and behavior change.* New York: John Wiley & Sons.

Kenny, C.B. (1989). *The field of play: A guide for the theory and practice of music therapy.* Atascadero, CA: Ridgeview Publishing Company.

Kiesler, D.J. (1983). *The paradigm shift in psychotherapy process research.* Paper presented at the National Institute of Mental Health Workshop on Psychotherapy Process Research, Bethesda-MD.

Langenberg, M., Frommer, J., & Tress, W. (1992). Qualitative Methodik zur Beschreibung und Interpretation musiktherapeutischer Behandlungswerke. *Musiktherapeutische Umschau, 4,* 258-278.

Langenberg, M., Frommer, J. & Tress, W. (1993). A qualitative research approach to analytical music therapy. *Music Therapy, 12*(1), 59-84.

Langenberg, M., Frommer, J. & Tress, W. (1995). From isolation to bonding: A music therapy case study of a patient with chronic migraines. *The Arts in Psychotherapy, 22,* 87-101.

Lincoln, Y. & Guba, E. (1985). *Naturalistic inquiry*. London: Sage.

Maso, I. (1989). *Kwalitatief onderzoek*. Meppel: Boom.

Meschede, H.G., Bender, W. & Pfeiffer H. (1983). Musiktherapie mit psychiatrischen problempatienten. *Psychotherapie und Medizinische Psychologie, 33*, 101-106.

Miles, M.B. & Huberman, A.M. (1984). *Qualitative data analysis: A sourcebook of new methods*. London: Sage.

Osborne, J.W. (1989). A phenomenological investigation of the musical representation of extra-musical ideas. *Journal of Phenomenological Psychology, 20*(2), 151-175.

Remmert, C. (1992). Wirkungsforschung in der musiktherapie: Ein beispiel teil I. *Musik-, Tanz-, und Kunsttherapie, 3*, 125-128.

Smeijsters, H. (1991). *Methoden van onderzoek in de muziektherapie en andere kreatieve therapieën*. Nijmegen: Hogeschool Nijmegen.

Smeijsters, H. (1993). Music therapy and psychotherapy. *The Arts in Psychotherapy, 20*, 223-229.

Smeijsters, H. (1995) Handboek muziektherapie. Heerlen, Netherlands: Melos.

Smeijsters, H. & van den Hurk, J. (1993a). Praktijkgericht onderzoek in de muziektherapeutische behandeling van een cliënte met kenmerken van anorexia nervosa. *Tijdschrift voor Kreatieve Therapie, 12*(1), 2-10.

Smeijsters, H. & J. van den Hurk (1993b). Research in practice in the music therapeutic treatment of a client with symptoms of anorexia nervosa. In M. Heal & T. Wigram (Eds.), *Music therapy in health and education*. London: Jessica Kingsley.

Smeijsters, H. & van den Hurk, J. (1994). Praxisorientierte forschung in der musiktherapie. *Musiktherapeutische Umschau, 15*(1), 25-42.

Smeijsters, H. & van den Berk, P. (1994). Music therapy with a client suffering from musicogenic epilepsy. A practice orientated qualitative single-case research. In *Proceedings of the Third European Arts Therapies Conference in Ferrara, volume 4.*

Smeijsters, H. & Rogers, P. (1993). *European music therapy research register.* Utrecht: Werkgroep Onderzoek Muziektherapie NVKT.

Strauss, A. & Corbin, J. (1990). *Basics of qualitative research: Grounded theory procedures and techniques.* London: Sage.

Strupp, H.H. (1990). The case of Helen R. *Psychotherapy, 27,* 644-656.

Tüpker, R. (1990). Wissenschaftlichkeit in kunsttherapeutischer forschung. *Musiktherapeutische Umschau, 11,* 7-20.

Yin, R.K. (1989). *Case study research. Design and methods.* London: Sage.

Translation: Dave Herman.

The Story of the Field of Play

Carolyn Bereznak Kenny

A story is in the telling and hearing. Literature is in the writing and reading. This is a story. I'm writing it down because Chief Simon Baker, elder of the Squamish Nation is telling us: "Write it down." He knows that oral traditions can die. But I'm also telling in the hope that you are hearing the story between the lines of what you are reading. We want to live so that others who walk along this path will be hearing and telling these stories, and so that they make new stories too.

When my colleague, Mechtild Langenberg, invited me to participate in the First International Symposium on Qualitative Research in Music Therapy, I decided that this occasion would be a good opportunity to elaborate on "The Story" of my research, particularly on the process of story making. Of the six presenters and twenty-five participants at the Symposium in Düsseldorf, many had read the works I had written about "The Field of Play," a theoretical approach which had emerged from a serious reflection of the way we describe our clinical work in music therapy. We had done the writing and reading. This was an opportunity for telling and hearing.

So at the Symposium, I presented a set of fragments about the story making process. The symposium members were part of my community. We have a shared knowledge. This was a time to delve deeper; to discover something significant about the way we work. It was a discursive and dialogical possibility.

The following points are an attempt to describe the story making process. I present myself to my colleagues as an impressionistic scene. Together we will construct a reality, a world, in this case, perhaps a research approach, which makes sense, given our shared experience in the field. I have chose to punctuate this monologue by numbers for the convenience of my responding colleagues, in the philosophical style of discourse and in the spirit of "fragments" of thought.

(1) The Story has always been a fascination for me. I tend toward myth. *The Mythic Artery* (Kenny, 1982), my first book, was an exploration of the creation stories of patients. It was a description of how, through my eyes, they seemed to spontaneously discover mythological themes without direction or guidance at times when they were hospitalized, in a state of chaos, confusion or illness. They needed healing and direction. It seemed that music must have presented abstract patterns to them which suggested mythological processes.

(2) In *The Field of Play* (Kenny, 1987; 1989) I felt pressed to articulate the structure of this mythological experience. We need these kinds of conceptual and theoretical tools to help us to understand and guide the experience. In the field of play, I discovered more than a structure. I came to the idea that the direct experience of music therapy, for me, was an experience of intense beauty in a heightened state of awareness. I further discovered that each person is a whole and complete form of beauty in my eyes. This left me free to describe the process of expansion, growth, change.

Some people do not understand how intimately my perception is connected to my cultural roots. Beauty is an important concept in the experience of aboriginal peoples. The creation of beauty is necessary for the continuity of life.

2.1) I take heart in one of the Navaho Blessing Way prayers:

> With beauty before me, I walk
> With beauty behind me, I walk
> With beauty above me, I walk
> With beauty below me, I walk
> From the East beauty has been restored
> From the South beauty has been restored
> From the West beauty has been restored
> From the North beauty has been restored
> From the zenith in the sky beauty has been restored
> From the nadir of the earth beauty has been restored
> From all around me beauty has been restored.

(3) In my twenty-five years of experience in music therapy, I have met many patients and clients who some would call "ugly": psychotic and crazy, demonstrating bizarre behavior; suffering and disturbed, coping with death; depressed and apathetic, full of sorrow; physically disfigured and challenged, difficult to behold.

(4) When I first met Debbie, so many years ago, many considered her to be grotesque: she was a quadriplegic; her face was severely disfigured; she drooled incessantly; she was nourished by a nasal/gastral tube; and she made bizarre sounds yet would not or could not speak. Yet I was inextricably attracted to her, to work with her in music therapy.

Many objected and said she was a hopeless case. Why waste your professional time? I was asked. There was no assuaging me. Debbie and I would find our worlds in the sound.

So we began a relationship which lasted for two years. Debbie had been in a terrible accident and within thirty seconds had gone from a vital, energetic young woman, wife, and mother of two children, into what some would describe as barely vegetable. As I got to know Debbie through our work in music therapy, I learned that, in fact, we had many similar conditions. We were both Native American. We each had two children, one girl and one boy. And in the sound we found our world. The staff began to comment, after a while, that we were starting to look like sisters when we smiled.

However, Debbie had some conditions which I did not. She had been traumatized physically, emotionally, psychologically, and spiritually. She must create a new life, which she expressed in our shared world.

There were many frustrating and difficult moments in the work with Debbie. In addition, in the hospital where we worked I was surrounded by death. I also was going through a difficult time in my personal life. So that one day it all seemed so hard that I looked at the drooling Debbie and the burning question presented itself: Why am I doing this? The answer was clear: For the Beauty.

My experience with Debbie, however difficult, was often permeated by a sense of beauty. This beauty had a rhythm and a form. Initially, I experienced her as a form of beauty, whole and complete. As our relationship began to develop in the sound the beauty would ebb and flow, open and close. I began to notice that these modes of engagement were similar to my other experiences of music therapy over the years; they were also similar to my experiences in the Longhouse of the

Musqueam people of the Salish nation during healing ceremonies, the Salish Guardian Spirit Dance Ceremonials. It didn't matter whether we called it therapy or healing. It was so human, so rich, so real.

Debbie and I had a life and I had to find a way of honoring our experience together by telling the truth. Writing about her progress in quantifiable language on charts became meaningless. I was using a language which was sedimented with values which were not mine and certainly did not accurately express my experiences with Debbie.

As a music therapist in the psychiatric unit of a large medical teaching hospital I had these feelings about "charting" in the past. But my professional identity urged me to comply. Older and wiser by the time Debbie and I met, I had written in hundreds of charts, enough to realize that this ritual was actually a killing thing. It encouraged standardization of patients. What did it kill? The human spirit. Individuality. The language was built around compliance to a set of social norms. It was built for control.

Debbie and I were equals. I had no desire to dominate her. We were both forms of beauty. Some of our human conditions were alike, some were different. In the therapy there was an exchange. In a sense, Debbie taught me to laugh; I taught her to play. Her first word after two years of silence was "piano" with no prompting from me. It was a surprise.

The birth of my burning question in the presence of my patient/friend triggered development of a theoretical approach which described our direct experience in music therapy. This approach is based on a personal encounter over time.

It is not a theory in the positivistic school. The research which emerged called the question: Was I willing to speak the truth? Could I behave in a professional environment with integrity? What meant more to me: my experience with patients like Debbie or the approval of my colleagues? Many of the latter believed we should not be concerned with description of our experience but rather with quantification and proof.

(5) Positivism is an organized method for combining deductive logic with precise empirical observations of individual behavior in order to discover and confirm a set of probabilistic causal laws that can be used to predict general patterns of human activity.

(6) In the guidelines for our symposium, Mechtild Langenberg stated: "We are more concerned with how to do research in music therapy and how to evaluate it than with the actual results."

(7) In order to move beyond the positivistic tendency for results, for proof, we build a community of researchers who can tell the more intimate nuances of the research story. This way we create a shared reality.

(8) In the philosophy and theory of science we have choices in our modes of research. Although positivism may still represent the received view through a pervasive presence in research studies, it is by no means the only view. And its presence may be more well known in some cultures of inquiry than in others. By "cultures of inquiry", I mean schools of thought, research traditions such as:

> comparative/historical
> ethnographic
> phenomenological
> hermeneutic
> theoretical
> empirical/analytical
> action
> evaluation.

Research in music therapy can be conducted in any of these categories. And, in fact, the more categories the better to shine light on to the research story.

(9) Qualitative research, the topic of our current meeting, can influence and be a part of any of the cultures of inquiry. For each can address the question of quality of experience, quality of life.

(10) Taylor and Bogdan (1984) offer a simple and useful description of qualitative research, with sweeping brush stokes and broad and encompassing categories. They state that, in general, quantitative research tends toward a positivistic mode and qualitative research tends toward the phenomenological mode. If we are serious about qualitative research as colleagues we can support and challenge each other by

screening out the last remnants of the positivistic view, particularly language, concepts, assumptions, values, accommodations of various kinds to the old approach, such as proving and cause and effect. Can we identify ourselves as qualitative researchers? Can we create from this place? These are central questions. We must be clear about which category we are functioning in and have a commitment to it. When we claim our place, there can be a more productive dialogue among ourselves and with others who hold different world views.

(11) Qualitative methodology refers in the broadest sense to research that produces descriptive data such as people's own written or spoken words and observable behavior. It is a way of approaching the empirical world (the world of experience), unlike the larger phenomenology, which can also approach non-observable behavior and an un-empirical world.

(12) Taylor & Bogdan (1984) describe qualitative research as inductive and holistic, naturalistic and non-intrusive. Qualitative researchers like to view things as if they were happening for the first time. They suspend judgement and consider diverse perspectives. Their validity criteria are based on first hand experience of life, unmediated through concepts, definitions and rating scales. Qualitative research is more of a craft.

(13) As qualitative researchers, we owe it to our readers to describe our methodology, the story of our approach. This is important because qualitative research does not offer a strict and standard set of methods, but rather guidelines which allow the research to stay vital and creative. We cannot assume a common understanding of our approach. This is an ethical issue. We offer this information as we can, when we can, as much as we can, depending on our own level of development, insight, and understanding. It is a developmental process in articulation.

(14) Most qualitative researchers, given the above characteristics of the approach, come up against the "category" problem. How do we organize our thoughts in such a referential totality? If we recognize the fact that we can never name all the conditions, all the variables, nor can we impose a reality onto context, how do we come to terms with the complexity and begin to organize our thoughts? This problem reveals why many researchers choose a positivistic approach. It seems to offer a less complex reality.

(15) In the story, the forms are not fixed or static, but dynamic. They move with the elements of the context. The story is a referential totality, a holistic approach. It keeps "sense." It makes sense. It moves.

(16) Qualitative research offers guidelines and, informed by these guidelines, many researchers have created methods.

(17) Phenomenology is a broad school of thought, philosophical in nature, from which a qualitative approach can emerge. Because of its philosophical nature, phenomenology does not always tend toward method. In fact, on philosophical grounds, the phenomenologist often rejects method entirely.

> 17.1) Although my own research is qualitative, in this sense, it is more phenomenological, more philosophical in tone. It barely stops short of categories, which are explicitly and concretely defined in the material world. My categories are more abstract, not so concrete. Although I create categories, I also resist. Although I define, I am, as well, repelled by definitions, attempting to embed ambiguity, leaving room for life.

(18) With the idea of grasping the eidos, or pure essence, of the direct experience of music therapy in its primordial form, I set out from non-empirical intuitions that do not apprehend sensory existence but focus rather on the intuition of imaginative order. This notion was presented by Edmund Husserl as "free phantasie variation."

> 18.1) Briefly, the free phantasie variation incorporates what Husserl calls exemplary intuition, imaginative repetition, and synthesis. The goal of this process is to identify essential elements which are found through essential intuition.

> 18.2) Often it takes the form of the telling of many stories about the same situation, or similar situations, in this case music therapy sessions. Narrative forms are produced repetitively until the eidos is discovered, shining through as the common elements in all the stories. The question is what are the recurring themes, which keep showing up in the story through many variations?

18.3) I wrote many such stories. Although I had reflected and wrote about my experiences with many patients and clients throughout the years, including Debbie, with whom my burning question seemed to take shape, I designed my dissertation study around my clinical experience with Jack. I wrote many descriptions of one session with Jack, beginning with the transcript from our session. From these descriptions, the seven fields in *The Field of Play* emerged.

18.4) It is essential to emphasize that the eidos, or essential elements, discovered in this process by the clinician-researcher relate only to the clinician-researcher; they reflect her view/interpretation of the experience with the client, her values and beliefs, including various spheres of influence, such as culture. We cannot assume that this eidos is universal, or even have the audacity to imagine that we can assume that the client has our same way of knowing and perceiving. This is about the reality of the clinician-researcher—an articulation, a revelation perhaps. We can assume or hope that our reality, in some way, influences that of the client's if we are in relation.

18.5) The eidos, in this case, is an articulation of the pure essence of my own experience with hundreds of patients and clients over time. Simultaneously, I long for "the other," a sense of the pure essence of my clients. Then there can be an exchange. In the music therapy, this might be experienced through authentic sounds, expressions of their human conditions.

19) A method could not reconstruct my experience in the music therapy with Debbie or Jack or Susan or others. I could not communicate our story in a method, per se, nor could I invent any method which could do this. But approaching the research task phenomenologically through free phantasie variation, I could tell the story in an imaginative way, staying close enough to our experience to still be art. I could hope to communicate the essence of the experience to others, thus offering a template of the referential totality, looking not for "facts" or causes or effects or proof, but rather for experience and meaning in an aesthetic and philosophical approach.

19.1) Consciousness is vast. Paradoxically, I revolt against method, but I uncover assumptions, discover principles, formulate concepts, create constructs so that my mind can comprehend what is going on in our experience, come to terms with it, accept it as fitting into a reality.

19.2) When a paradox exists, perhaps it is best to embrace, articulate, and elaborate upon its elements rather than avoid them. In this way, we can stretch possibilities in the philosophy and theory of science, eventually offering greater possibilities to patients and clients by increasing the scope and range of practice and research. When there is truly paradox, then paradox must be included in the construction of the story and be integral to it. My focus on "The Story" would not preclude my interest in, although perhaps not fascination with, "hard" data.

(20) One of Husserl's greatest contributions was the discovery and elaboration of the "intentionality of experience." He realized that in a pervasive sense, the world is our construction. It is therefore important to study our worldviews.

20.1) Can I comment on the worldview of the patient with any confidence? The answer is no. In Debbie's case, she only began to speak after two years of music therapy. For two years, the musical language was what we had. We also had a relationship which embraced both our world views. I could articulate mine verbally. I had to sense hers.

Debbie communicated her worldview to me non-verbally through her music, her presence, her many forms of communication, through her heart.

We loved. We cared. We created together in the sound. In the Field of Play, when I become overwhelmed by the complexity, I remember that in this theory there is at the core one simple idea. This is a field of loving and creating.

(21) In this way, any theory is a self-study of the theorist, as well as the theorist's spheres of influence, culture being one, clients themselves being another. This is *The Field of Play*.

(22) It is a story, seen through the eyes of the beholder. It is fiction. Theodor Adorno (1982) comments on Husserl's phenomenology: "Hence if anyone loves a paradox, he can really say with strict truth if he will allow for ambiguity, that the element which makes up the life of phenomenology as of all 'eidedit' science is 'fiction'" (p. 198). For Adorno, there is no doubt about the fictional character of phenomenology. He articulates "fiction" as the keystone of the approach.

(23) The next step in the pursuit of knowledge and creation is the dialogue with trusted colleagues who share a similar knowledge base, a similar experience, as suggested by Thomas Kuhn. This is the creation story of the knowledge of a field.

(24) One of the important aspects of Husserl's work, for music therapists and music therapy researchers, is that we can remain in art yet dwell in science which is clearly not positivistic. Perhaps fiction communicates the depth of our lived experience. How can we prove a sense of wonder, psychological pain, release, or imagine that it could be measured in some objective reality? These human experiences happen relationally, in a shared reality, a shared subjectivity, experienced by both patient and therapist.

(25) Through his method of free phantasie variation we gather comparative fiction, elaborated, according to Husserl, through imaginative stages of intuitional ideation. Then we compare and contrast our stories of lived experience in music therapy.

(26) Adorno, like Husserl, was concerned about method in studies of human experience, particularly aesthetic experience. He said that "method must constantly do violence to unfamiliar things, though it exists only so that they may be known. It must model itself after the other" (p. 12). In other words, there is an integrity between the experience and the method. Yet in this case, knowledge, as method, creates sorrow because it takes us away from, even does violence to, experience.

(27) In music therapy, the closer our methods are to art the more integrity they possesses. This provides more opportunities for communicating direct experience, for describing it, learning about it, understand-

ing it, responding to it. After all, what is research for if not to learn and to understand, to improve and to change, to grow?

27.1) Indeed Adorno (1982) takes a radical approach to any who would propose an objective reality which assumes a first principle or absolute position. He says that "by furnishing the principle from which all being proceeds, the subject promotes itself. . . . They use their subjectivity to subtract the subject from truth and their idea of objectivity is as a residue" (pp. 14-15).

27.2) Those of us who have used positivistic methods in our work shudder at the thought. But Adorno, above all else, inspires us to acknowledge and specify our various "subjectivities" so that they are not embedded in our objectivity as implied truth. Is there a sanctity to our methods? Is science a religion after all? Can we placidly accept norms, which become so embedded, that they go virtually unchallenged and uncritiqued?

27.3) Perhaps we can consider the developmental process of the life of the researcher. For the first five years of my work, I did only clinical practice. From then I worked as a clinician/researcher. After the first five years of my work life, I was interested in proving my effectiveness as a music therapist and in proving the effectiveness of music therapy as a field. I talked to people about it. I soul-searched. Am I doing the right thing? Is music therapy the variable that is making the difference? During this five-ten year period, I was looking for effectiveness in my research, hoping to prove that music therapy worked. During the period from ten to fifteen years into my work life, I turned more toward historical reflection on ancient healing systems, description of clinical work, and the comparison of ancient tribal and contemporary systems. Fifteen to twenty years into my working life I focused on phenomenological/theoretical research. Now in my twenty-fifth year, I would describe my research as aesthetic, the story of the work and how it relates to life as a whole.

(28) Feyerabend (1975), in an equally radical position, when consider-

ing issues of epistemology, presents an anarchist theory of knowledge. He says: "Science is an essentially anarchistic enterprise: theoretical anarchism is more humanitarian and more likely to encourage progress than its law-and-order alternative" (p. 9).

28.1) In an interesting summary of a portion of his approach, he reveals the story, the myth, the fiction of science:

> Thus science is much closer to myth than a scientific philosophy is prepared to admit. It is one of the many forms of thought that have been developed by man, and not necessarily the best. It is conspicuous, noisy, and impudent, but it is inherently superior only for those who have already decided in favour of a certain ideology, or who have accepted it without having ever examined its advantages and its limits. And as the accepting and rejecting of ideologies should be left to the individual it follows that the separation of state and church must be supplemented by the separation of state and science, that most recent, most aggressive, and most dogmatic religious institution. Such a separation may be our only change to achieve a humanity we are capable of, but have never fully realized. (p.238)

28.2) Feyerabend's passionate critique of ways of knowing and ways of proving also might place us in a shudder, at least those of us who still want to believe in science in some form. The question is: Are we inside or outside science? For those of us who choose to stay inside, if merely at the inner edge, perhaps our despair is assuaged by the possibility of change within—something like Thomas Kuhn's revolution.

28.3) Consider how the "burden of proof" ideology influences and determines clinical services, research budgets, policy. If the received view, much less the broader scientific view, is the only view, how does this limit our ways of knowing, of discovering, of providing? Feyerabend challenges the moral high ground of a limited reality. How can we assume that the "burden of proof" approach is better than an approach founded on accumulating evidence and/or anecdotal reports (stories), especially when it comes to phenomena such as emotion, expression, anger, love. Again, we cannot assume that a single tradition is the only tradition, or the best. These movements are contextual and complexly derived.

(29) This begs the question of the purpose of research. In the two hundred-year-old battle between the natural sciences and the behavioral, psychological, and social sciences, what can we honestly say that we can prove? What are the missing steps between philosophy and research in our field? Have we articulated a philosophy (which must always be at the root of theory and research)? Perhaps our purpose is to create guidelines for the practitioner, a way to reflect on the process as we grow and change.

THEORETICAL NARRATIVE

(30) The following is one of the narrative descriptions created in my process of free phantasie variation. I offer it to you here, because it is the one colleagues have focused on and critiqued most productively:[1]

The first important step in *The Field of Play* is the acknowledgment of an aesthetic. An aesthetic is a field or environment containing conditions for the creation of beauty. In the music therapy experience the human person is an aesthetic and thus an environment of being and acting through relationship and music, with a particular attention for human growth and development. As an aesthetic, the human person holds love as an informing energy which provides conditions in the field.

The process in the field of the aesthetic has to do with changing places acknowledged and developed through musical experience. The field of the aesthetic is a place which appreciates what is present, yet has an anticipation for and belief in what is possible in the emerging moment, all this in reference to learning, growth and change. It has to do with stretching the boundaries of what we consider our limitations—for client and therapist. The aesthetic forms a defined, yet open space; one which provides safety and support, one which receives all being and acting as part of the ongoing process of change (defined through the emerging

---

[1] The material in comment #30 is from Kenny, 1987, pp. 100-108.

relationship between client and therapist).

Anticipation is another important condition in this field. The therapist is committed to maintaining a posture which waits enduringly for the slightest micromovement, sound or pattern indicative of a movement toward wholeness. This movement could be dramatic or subtle. These movements are initiated by the client although they may be inspired by the therapist. Movements toward wholeness reflect the logic of the self-organizing system. The therapist notices, receives and responds to this movement, signified by the patterns and textures of sound. If the patient is willing to share, that is, not only express, but also communicate this changing process, a step has been taken toward communication, relationship and rehabilitation.

Fundamentally, the therapist is limited in terms of what s/he is able or willing to notice. But it is hoped that through her own human experience and skill, she will notice and respond to some significant aspect of the patient's stretching boundaries in the direction of positive change.

The field also resonates in many domains and dimensions. For example, even though it is moving toward emotions in its primary intention it has effects in the cognitive and sensori-motor areas as well. All expressions are received, acknowledged and valued.

Each aesthetic is highly individualized and never value-free. Values or beliefs, even though they may be nonverbal, constitute conditions in the field. In the aesthetic of the therapist, the following values and thus conditions are present—they form a foundation for all seven fields:

(1) Value for a particular form of beauty, which has to do with changing places particularly in human growth, development and learning, feelings of expansion, feelings of appreciation for all the variables in the field (including attitudes, beliefs, behaviors, observers, light, extra sound, etc.) inclusively, openness.

(2) Value for an existential approach which views each moment as the only moment in time in the given field.

(3) Belief in the principles of the self-organizing system—that each human being is unique and that part of each human, no matter how deeply traumatized, holds the most logical and effective plan for the whole of her development, as well as each step in the sequence of development and change.

In the final analysis, the aesthetic represents a way of being which carries information and conditions. It stresses the importance of subtle, non-verbal cues communicated before the onset of concrete activity. It represents the sum total of who we are, and transmits information about who we are on a subtle level before the onset of relationship. Being "who we are" communicates a field of being and establishes conditions to which clients respond during improvisation. The conditions of the aesthetic also grant support and permission for particular parts of the client to emerge and evolve within the musical space and the field of play.

When the aesthetics of client and therapist overlap, that which is able to come forth and create a relational field emerges. Once again, the logic of a natural self-organization is in play. A commitment is made to this new field when there is a point of engagement in the musical gestures. This new field is called the musical space. It is a space which is closed, i.e., a private space which is reserved only for therapist and client. The musical improvisation is the meeting place between the abstract and the concrete. It represents abstract phenomena such as ideas, emotions, attitudes, etc., yet is a sensorial phenomenon in sound forms.

In the musical space, the client and therapist merge into a pool of human expression and communication. They become equally significant participants and formers of the being and an acting in this new field though relationship of the two. The participants create this space through their relationship to each other represented in the music. The playing of music is a developmental action and represents whatever each selects to place into the field of the musical space, once again demonstrating organization. The commitment to play music together is the most consistent and reliable condition in this field.

The environment which was first formed by the aesthetic is now realized through the musical space. The music, as created by client and therapist together form the space just as the aesthetic previously formed the space prior to the engaging activity between therapist and client. Therapist and client come together in the creative act of making music.

The musical space is a self-contained safety zone which develops out of the relationship between the two participants. This relationship, which becomes contained in a mutually created space now becomes the most formative condition in the field.

Once the trust has been established in the musical space and the participants have developed a relationship through sound which creates a home base or constant, it is then possible for the musical space to expand into the field of play.

The field of play is a new field, one which includes the aesthetics and the musical space. It grows out of these two, yet expands into a field of experimentation, play and modeling. It is an open space, which is more conducive to innovation and more fluid in nature.

Each participant plays and models forms which hold meaning for the individual creating the sound. The client improvises and searches for meaningful patterns and sounds. The therapist follows the patterns and forms of the client to intensify the texture—to explore and develop the feelings or thought within the improvisational form. Similarly, the therapist presents models of meaningful sounds which s/he determines may be useful to the client from her experience. When a pattern or form is intuitively embraced by client, therapist or both, the assumption is that this form holds meaning for the client and/or therapist and therefore will be played or developed for a while—to investigate meaning, communication, expression, growth.

Through this relationship of play and modeling within the musical improvisation, each selects the pieces or parts or wholes of musical patterning which make sense in the authentic expression of the self and in the mutually creative process. Again, this is a form of organizing sound.

Hopefully, the openness of the aesthetics and the trust developed in the musical space continues to function in the field of play as therapist and client engage in spontaneous playing with patterns, rhythms and sounds, harmonics and melodies, consonance and dissonance, dynamics, etc. The assumption is that authentic sounds will emerge and provide the starting point for development. Most often these authentic expressions have to do with deep emotions, which for whatever reason, are inexpressible in verbal language. The expression and communication of these emotions initiates growth and change.

It is believed that within the process of the musical improvisation development will occur. The process is the product.

The field of play contains four interactive elements or fields: ritual, a particular state of consciousness, power, and creative process. These fields overlap to also create conditions and relationships which develop the potential of the field of play over time.

Ritual is the set of repeatable forms created through the conditions present at the time of the session. These forms can include the overall form of the session itself and all of the musical forms expressed in the musical improvisation, and any other pattern which is repeated in the ritual space. The actual playing of music is a constant. The circumstances are reliable, replicable and constant—the room, entering the room and greetings, the action of verbal and musical dialogue, moments of silence and stopping, playing again through several progressions, endings, good-byes.

Hopefully, the ritual forms, which emerge organically from the experience, particularly in the musical improvisation itself, will provide, as the musical space does, another ground base. This field of support allows the participants to try out innovation within the security of constants or within the framework of the repeatable forms which have emerged in the field of play thus far.

The most important condition in this field, then, is the condition of constants. Once again, this emerging structure demonstrates a tendency to organize through identifying these constants in the field. Once again ritual interplays with the aesthetic, the musical space and the field of play, representing an organic process.

A particular state of consciousness is a field of focused relaxation and intense concentration, yet playfulness. Once again, it is a state between the abstract and the concrete and thus bridges two realities. One is aware of feelings and thought yet also engaged in the sensorial realm of creation of sound forms. This creation assumes an ability to select and screen input aesthetically as it is presented through the results of musical improvisation. Some sound patterns and forms are accepted, some are rejected, depending on their success or failure as authentic expressions.

In this state of consciousness one is self-motivated. It is a motivational state which plays itself into change through musical form. It thus reflects another type of organization and also includes all previous fields and conditions. It is an open field which allows one to travel in the dimension of consciousness into a fluid reality which is not contingent on circumstance, e.g., disability. The most outstanding condition in this field is the state itself.

Power is a phenomenon which sets the patient in motion. It represents the field which is created through a relationship between will and receptivity which yields inner motivation and action. It is critical to human growth and development and essential for change. If the patient has been favorably inclined toward the previous elements, the particular state of consciousness has prepared him or her for the inner motivation, the ritual would have given him or her the ground base needed for experimentation, and s/he has gathered and continues to gather substance through the ongoing musical space and the field of play. Therefore it is possible to allow interaction between the state of inner motivation and receptivity in order to actualize power.

Power is a contained phenomenon and is associated also with the accumulation of enough energy to initiate change. Therefore it is a threshold point. It builds over time until there is a natural breakthrough. In the musical form, it is most easily recognized through initiation of expression and assertiveness on the part of the client. The most important condition in this field is actualization so that the client can experience the concrete results of his musical gestures, hear his/her own power in this movement and thus maintain an ongoing feeding of the state of inner motivation and receptivity to new forms.

Creative process is the last field in the model. It is a result of the interplay among all the previous elements, yet it is the process itself as well as the product. The process is field-creating but also self-creating or self-actualizing. It is organic, emerging sequentially from each previous influence and existential, proceeding from and to each moment in time. This is demonstrated in patterns of sound or receptivity to sound in the experience. This is the holistic and organic nature of the field.

(31) This is one of the descriptions and perhaps it is the most abstract. It is theoretical in nature. Other variations include, the transcript of the session, a concrete description of the music therapy session, or an empirical narrative description of the session.

> 31.1) From the narratives, certain definitions were discovered and offered to a panel of seven members, along with a videotape of the session and other descriptive materials. Panel members were asked to answer a questionnaire. Collectively, more variations were produced in the research community in the initial study. Over the last ten years, since the concept began, the material has been shared with clinicians and social scientists. So collective variations continue to be produced.

> 31.2) In my dialogues with colleagues, most people have an easy enough time understanding two of the seven modes of engagement in the Field of Play: the musical space and the field of

play. Some have hypothesized that this is because they recognize them as possible metaphors from psychoanalytic theory, particularly Winnicott. Others can understand the first mode of engagement, the aesthetic, particularly clinicians who have done a lot of clinical musical improvisation. However, the last four modes of engagement, the ones which stem clearly from my Native American worldview, are difficult for many. Some have fragmented associations. Some perceive a different order. Some reject entirely. With the last four—ritual, a particular state of consciousness, power and creative process—I see the healing ceremonies in the Longhouse. I see this happening with my clients and patients too. The Longhouse is in play. It is not an objective reality, rather a memory, which is etched into my perceptual field. It is a way of interpreting experience, which we could say is culturally derived. It is the story of who I am, where I have come from, my roots, where I belong. These memories help to form and shape my experience. If there are universal elements, they emerge from the dialogue with colleagues whom I respect and can trust to reveal myself, in the sharing of human stories.

(32) Some moments are epiphany for me in my experience with clients. I can sense change. I can sense birth, just like in the initiation ceremonies in the Longhouse, initiation to be reborn out of dis-ease. I cannot compromise these moments with Debbie, who represented hundreds of other patients and clients over twenty-five years of practice, with language which is a lie. The question is: What is our language as a field, as a culture? Stories of real life experience are not lies. They are full descriptions which communicate the richness of life. They present possible worlds. These were moments of intense beauty in a heightened state of awareness. In a sense, they are beyond words. But we try to communicate them anyway, in our research and to honor the traditions of the culture of science.

(33) Beauty counts for humans. I am reassured when Herbert Marcuse (1962) says: "The analysis of the cognitive function of phantasy is thus led to aesthetics as the 'science of beauty', behind the aesthetic form lies the repressed harmony of sensuousness and reason" (p. 130).

CONCLUSION

In our intellectual time, amidst the despair and disillusionment expressed in post-modern thought, we enact our intellectual pursuits within a tradition of deconstructing and constructing, to make sense out of contemporary life, to build something grounded in tradition, yet responsive to our modern conditions of life. What rises out of the ash? What new ideas, new approaches, new forms can be? What is our story now? And, What can and will it be?

Those of us in a position of responsibility must dream. We must imagine a new reality, connected to the old, yet living in the new. And we must create a vision to guide us into the future too.

This is our story as a field.

When we discussed our spheres of influence at the Symposium amidst the process of constructing creation stories, we acknowledged the central role of cultural influence. This is a difficult influence to articulate, because culture is essentially implied. Only when we compare, can we see, name, articulate what it is. How does culture affect our ways of knowing, our ways of thinking, our ways of creating?

My colleagues, in the final moments, challenged me to say more about the influence of my Native American roots on my ways of thinking about things, about *The Field of Play* and other works.

Although I have been socialized to the ways of knowing of the dominant society and can be in them and enjoy them, I often feel alone and alienated. Only when I am with Native peoples do I feel truly at home about knowing. It seems that, collectively, we know things, which remain unspoken, yet exist. There is a recognition of like-mindedness, a feeling of belonging. This is familiar and nurturing to me, not only intellectually, but spiritually and it also effects my physical being, because I feel at home. This way of knowing is strong and clear. It holds us together as a people. It is the way we see, the way we judge, the way we determine what is real, what is important. This comforts me. I know who I am.

That is not to say that all people of aboriginal descent always think about things in the same way. However, I experience a similarity, amongst my friends from different bands and tribes, which constitutes a consensus in what I would call core spiritual beliefs which are reflected, perhaps in different ways, in each group. They are reflected as values and subsequently constructs and systems which guide daily life. Systems reflect values, which reflect beliefs. For example, traditionally, we can say that most Native peoples believe in an intimate connection between the people and the land. This affects the ways spaces are created in the community. One example is the creation of therapeutic, or healing, space.

In the Native American reality, there are specific ways of thinking about things which communicate value. These concepts emerge out of a profound dialogue between the sacred and the mundane. Traditional Native societies are built on spiritual values, enacted in daily life and creating lifestyle for Native peoples. Some of these concepts are:

The Story

Space

Beauty

Vision

Community

Intuition

The story is not merely an intellectual construct. It is a way of being in the moment. Often, stories are not written down, but rather embedded in memory through oral tradition. Because our worldview is intimately connected to the land, space emerges as central in our ways of thinking. This value is manifested through ceremonial space, which functions to maintain our culture, to prevent illness, to heal. Our connection to Nature is revealed in our value for Beauty. Beauty is a holistic reality, which includes spiritual, physical, emotional, cognitive and psychological aspects. Vision is a way of seeing and is linked to a value for particular states of consciousness, energy, spirit, the importance of the dream, traveling in an alternate reality to obtain resources for our groups in order to live a good life. Intuition is a way of knowing which could be called a sophisticated form of logic, which includes the senses, history. It is instant recognition. Community is who we are, where we have come from, where we are going. There is not a concept of a split-off self in the Native American reality. One exists as part of and on behalf of the others. The individual is only within the group, yet brings her uniqueness to the group. So there is an exchange, an honoring of both, all in relation, ancestors too.

REFERENCES

Adorno, T.W. (1982). *Against epistemology, a metacritique: Studies in Husserl and the phenomenological autonomies*. Oxford: Blackwell.

Astrov, M. (Ed). (1946). *The winged serpent: American Indian prose and poetry*. Boston: Beacon Press.

Berleant, A. (1970). *The aesthetic field: A phenomenology of aesthetic experience*. Springfield, Illinois: Charles C. Thomas.

Cassell, E.J. (1991). *The nature of suffering and the goals of medicine*. New York: Oxford University Press.

Coltelli, L. (1990). *Winged words: American Indian writers speak*. Lincoln: University of Nebraska Press.

Dissanayake, E. (1992). *Homo aestheticus: Where art comes from and why*. New York: The Free Press.

Eagleton, T. (1990). *The significance of theory*. Cambridge, MA: Basil Blackwell, Inc.

Feyerabend, P. (1975). *Against method: Outline of an anarchistic theory of knowledge*. London: NLB.

Flax, J. (1990). *Thinking fragments: Psychoanalysis, feminism, and postmodernism in the contemporary west*. Berkeley: University of California Press.

Husserl, E. (1952). *Ideas: General introduction to pure phenomenology*. New York: The Macmillan Company.

Husserl, E. (1964). *The idea of phenomenology*. The Hague: Martinus Nijhoff.

Husserl, E. (1964). *The Paris lectures*. The Hague: Martinus Nijhoff.

Husserl, E. (1965). *Phenomenology and the crisis of philosophy*. New York: Harper and Row.

Kenny, C. B. (1982). *The mythic artery: The magic of music therapy*. Atascadero, CA: Ridgeview Publishing Co.

Kenny, C. B. (1987). The field of play: A theoretical study of music therapy process. (Doctoral dissertation) Santa Barbara, CA: The Fielding Institute.

Kenny, C. B. (1989). *The field of play: A guide for the theory and practice of music therapy*. Atascadero, CA: Ridgeview Publishing Co.

Koestenbaum, P. (1978). *The new image of the person: The theory and practice of clinical philosophy*. Westport, CT: Greenwood Press.

Kuhn, T. (1962). *The structure of scientific revolutions*. Chicago, IL: The University of Chicago Press.

Marcuse, H. (1962). *Eros and civilization*. New York: Vintage Books.

Merleau-Ponty, M. (1973). *The prose of the world*. Evanston, IL: Northwestern University Press.

Morgan, G. (1983). *Beyond method*. Beverly Hills, CA: Sage.

O'Brien, M. and Little, C. (Eds.). (1990). *Reimaging American: The arts of social change*. Philadelphia, PA: New Society Publishers.

Sartre, J.P. (1963). *Essays in aesthetics*. New York: Philosophical Library.

Sartre, J.P. (1963). *Search for a method*. New York: Knopf.

Sartre, J.P. (1972). *The transcendence of the ego*. New York: Farrar, Strauss and Giroux.

Taylor, S.J. and Bogdan, R. (1984). *Introduction to qualitative research methods: The search for meanings*. New York: John Wiley and Sons.

Tesch, R. (1990). *Qualitative research: Analysis types and software tools*. New York: The Falmer Press.

Torgovnick, M. (1990). *Gone primitive: Savage intellects, modern lives*. Chicago: The University of Chicago Press.

MONOLOGUE 4

Authenticity Issues In Qualitative Research

Kenneth E. Bruscia

CONTEXT AND DEFINITION

Because qualitative research is a relatively new scientific endeavor, the development of standards to insure the integrity of an inquiry is still very much in process. Two works have contributed greatly to the topic.

In 1985, Lincoln and Guba proposed four standards for ensuring what they call the "trustworthiness" of a qualitative inquiry, each representing a corresponding requirement in positivistic research. An inquiry has *credibility* when its methodology is appropriate to the purpose of the study (which parallels internal validity in positivistic research). An inquiry has *transferability* when the findings are applicable to situations other than the original inquiry (which parallels external validity). It has *dependability* when the data and findings are obtained consistently (which parallels reliability). And an inquiry has *confirmability* when the findings can be confirmed by other researchers (which parallels objectivity).

Later, the same authors (Guba & Lincoln, 1989) added another four criteria aimed at ensuring the "authenticity" of an inquiry. They are:
1) *ontological* authenticity (when the inquiry leads to enlarged personal constructions); 2) *educative* authenticity (when the inquiry leads to improved understanding of the constructions of others); 3) *catalytic* authenticity (when the inquiry leads to action); and 4) *tactical* authenticity (when the inquiry empowers persons to act).

I would like to quickly establish that the authenticity issues and standards presented in this chapter have not arisen from the work of these authors; in fact, I have not found a discussion of them anywhere else in the literature. Rather, my ideas have emerged from my own personal struggles to be authentic as a researcher, and, to be perfectly honest, from the inauthenticity that I sometimes perceive in other researchers.

Authenticity has been described in great detail by existential philosophers and psychotherapists of this century, and although their ideas have influenced me greatly, I would like to offer my own definition of it specifically as it pertains to research: When I am authentic as a researcher, I bring into my awareness whatever is possible for me to bring into it regarding my study; I act in a way that is consistent with what is in my awareness; and, I take appropriate responsibility not only for what is and is not in my awareness, but also for what I do and do not do in relation to it.

This conceptualization of authenticity has two distinctive features: First, it is an *intra*subjective standard which governs the researcher's relationship to him/herself; it is not an *inter*subjective standard which governs relationships among the researcher, participant, phenomenon and scholarly community. Second, in my definition, authenticity is an ongoing *process* that a researcher goes through from the beginning of the research to its ultimate conclusion; it is not something to be evaluated after the study has been completed only in terms of its outcomes. For me, authenticity is not determined by the value of what I did after I did it—it is determined by *who* I am while I am doing whatever I do. Thus, authenticity, as defined here, is an ongoing process of taking responsibility for what is in one's own awareness regarding all aspects of the research.

I believe that this kind of authenticity is foundational to all other standards of integrity, and as such is a fundamental requirement for all qualitative researchers. How can I be trustworthy to other researchers if I cannot trust myself as one? And how can I trust myself if I do not take responsibility for what is in my awareness? How can I enlarge my constructions and the constructions of others if I am not aware of, or do not take responsibility for, what my constructions are as the one who is enlarging these constructions? And, how can my research lead others to insight, empowerment and action, if I am unable to achieve the same with regard to myself as a researcher?

The purpose of the present work is to examine the various authenticity issues that can arise at various stages of a qualitative inquiry, and in so doing, to propose standards for authenticity of intent, paradigm, focus, context, method, findings, and communication.

As we will discuss later, I do not regard this chapter as a research study; it is more of a personal narrative which describes my ideas about authenticity as a researcher, based upon informal and unsystematic observations of myself and other researchers and many hours of contemplation on the struggles with authenticity that I have encountered.

AUTHENTICITY OF INTENT

Am I Doing Research?

The first and most basic question of authenticity for a researcher is: Is it my intent to do *research*, and is that what I am actually doing? Or more personally, am I being a *researcher* when I am doing what I am doing?

This is a particularly challenging question because in the new paradigm, research has many different definitions and goals, and rather unclear boundaries. As a result, each researcher has to find his/her own answer to this question based on personal constructs of what is and what is not research.

Is it Research or Therapy?

Authenticity of intent is in particular jeopardy when researchers study their own clinical work, either as they are doing it or afterwards. The boundaries here are fuzzy indeed as evidenced by the number of reports which are purported to be clinical studies or qualitative research projects.

Research and therapy certainly have many similarities and areas of overlap, but it is essential to recognize that they are fundamentally different in both intent and outcome. When I work with a client as a therapist it is not the same as studying my work with a client as a researcher. For me, the intent of research is to gain insight for the scholarly community, whereas the intent of therapy is to help a specific client achieve a state of well-being. To be authentic, then, I must acknowledge that when I am doing research, my primary intent is scholarly rather than clinical; and when I am doing therapy my primary intent is clinical rather than scholarly. Moreover, when I attempt to do both at the same time, it may not be possible to pursue them with equal devotion. Ultimately, I may have to choose to do one at the risk of the other. Being authentic requires me to acknowledge this possibility and then take responsibility for the choices I make.

This is not to say that research and therapy do not both involve gaining insight—they do. However, the difference is that when I intend to do therapy, I seek insight for the client's sake not for the sake of other clients, other therapists, other researchers, or for the sake of insight itself. Thus, in therapy, insight is the means to an end, while in research it is an end in itself.

Going even further, in therapy, I am seeking only to expand *my* knowledge of the client and the *client's* knowledge of the client and me—I am not seeking to increase *your* knowledge (as reader) of us, or your knowledge of yourself as a therapist with your clients. Thus, studying my own clinical work to further inform my own work, and thereby improve its effectiveness, is different in intent from studying my own clinical work to inform you, the reader, about what I have discovered through my clinical work. The former is clinical work while the latter is research.

This distinction is particularly significant when comparing research with those aspects of the therapy process which involve gathering information, such as assessment and evaluation. When I *assess* the client as a therapist, my primary intent is to better understand the client and his/her needs so that I can better address those needs within the therapy process; when I assess the client as a researcher (or study my assessment of a client as a therapist), my primary intent is to better understand music therapy assessment itself while also discovering what implications my findings might have for others outside of the immediate clinical context. As a therapist, I assess the client as who s/he is; as a researcher, I study who the client is and my assessment of him/her as an example; as a therapist, the *primary* implications of my assessment are clinical and client-specific; as a researcher, the *primary* implications of my assessment are scholarly and context-specific.

The therapist says to the client: I want to understand you purely for your sake; the researcher says to the client/participant: I want to better understand you and my clinical understanding of you—if possible for your own sake but primarily for the sake of others. The therapist says to the reader of a clinical assessment: I hope that what I learned about this client will help you in working with him/her; a researcher says to the reader: I hope that what I learned about my client through assessment may benefit you as a therapist with your clients or researcher with your participants.

Similarly when I *evaluate* the effects of my work in the role of therapist, my primary intent is to discover whether a specific client is improving as the result of my efforts, for the sole purpose of enhancing the client's progress or my effectiveness. When I study the effectiveness of my work in the role of researcher, my intent is to demonstrate to myself and others outside of the clinical context what aspects of my work were effective or ineffective, and the implications they may have for other therapists and clients. Here again, a therapist's goals are clinical and client-specific, whereas as researcher's goals are scholarly and context-specific.

In clinical evaluation, the therapist says to a client: I want to evaluate your progress so that I can help you better; a researcher says to a client-participant: I want to evaluate your progress so that I and other therapists will have a better understanding of what works and does not work.

Notice that there are three tiers of insight found on the continuum between therapy and research: working directly with the client to understand the client and what will help him/her (a clinical pursuit); reflecting on my work with the client to better inform my efforts as a therapist with this client (a clinical pursuit); and meta-reflecting on my work as a therapist to increase understanding within the scholarly-therapeutic community (a research pursuit). Perhaps the first two clinical tiers involve searching for insights, and the third tier involves re-searching them.

Authenticity requires that when I do research, I acknowledge that I am doing it to enlighten and benefit first you and me as scholar/therapists—then future clients of ours as therapists, and when appropriate, the clients who provided the original data. It is important to mention at this point that clients who participate in a study can benefit from it only if they are ready for and capable of benefitting from the insights it brings; and when they are not ready, the findings can seriously endanger the therapeutic process. Needless to say, it is inauthentic (and unethical) to claim that a research study will be of direct benefit to client-participants when its potential effects on them are uncertain.

Given all of the above differences between therapy and research, authenticity also requires that I distinguish among the following activities: writing a clinical report (a confidential entry into the client's records or files), writing a clinical case study (a written description of my work with a client that is published), and case study research (a systematic inquiry into a particular clinical phenomenon as exemplified in my clinical work with a particular client).

Am I Inquiring or Disclosing?

Another snare for inauthenticity occurs when research is confused with expository writings, such as theoretical papers and personal narratives. A theoretical paper is different from a research report in several ways.

In strictest terms, a theory is speculative, it is not always or entirely based on findings from research or clinical practice, and in fact it can rarely be substantiated; in contrast, research is either deductive or inductive—it is always concerned with making sense out of a specific body of data gathered.

This distinction does not mean that a theory may not be the result of a research study. In fact, this is often the case in qualitative research. The main thing to keep in mind is that there is a real difference between a speculative theory which combines, relates and extends data and findings from many different research studies and practices, and an empirical theory which is based upon and grounded in data from one specific study.

Another big difference is that a speculative theory is usually an attempt to relate many different questions and problems within an entire phenomenal field, whereas an empirical theory focuses much more specifically on a particular question or problem within such a field. In short, speculative theories are broader in concern and wider in applicability than empirical theories.

Thus, for the sake of authenticity, I must be clear with myself as to when I am being speculative and when I am being empirical, when I am looking at an entire phenomenal field and when I am focusing on a part of it, and when the applicability of theory is broad and when it is narrow.

The second type of expository writing often confused with research is what I call a personal narrative—a paper which expresses the author's thoughts, feelings, beliefs and opinions on a particular topic, with little if any reference to data other than one's own experience. This type of writing is different from research because it is not a form of inquiry which involves focused and self-critical methods of gathering new data, but rather relies on the orderly communication of already experienced personal experiences. When I write something based on what is already in my experience, rather than on new data that I intentionally and systematically gather, then my intent is not to do research but to merely discuss and share with an audience what I am already thinking or contemplating.

Another difference is that a personal narrative is an elaboration of what is already known rather than an attempt to discover what is unknown. It seems obvious that the reason why a researcher begins an inquiry is because s/he is in a state of ignorance about something—not because s/he already knows it. In contrast, an author writes a personal narrative because s/he wants to share something and perhaps extend or speculate on something that is already in awareness. The former requires ignorance and discovery; the latter requires insight and elaboration. (I am often reminded of a professor who gave me some good advice when I was doing my doctoral dissertation: "A good researcher needs more ignorance than wisdom!").

Of course, some might argue that personal experience is a form of data, and that to gather data from oneself is a valid form of qualitative research. I agree to a certain extent, but if no distinctions are made, then everything that comes out of anyone's mouth can qualify as research— which to me is a very frightening prospect indeed! I think we can make the following distinctions:

* Self-expression without systematic inquiry (when I am not a researcher or a participant and express my views)

* Self as research participant (when I serve as one of the participants in my own study)

* Self-inquiry as researcher (when I study myself to clarify and perhaps bracket my contributions as researcher to the inquiry process)

* Self-inquiry as researcher and participant (when I study myself as the main participant). An example of this is what Moustakas (1990) calls heuristic inquiry.

With all of this said, I have two final comments. First, I would like to summarize the main requirements for research: there must be an inquiry into what is unknown, the inquiry must involve the systematic gathering of data, the inquiry must be self-monitored with regard to integrity, the findings must be context-specific in addition to being client-specific, and the results must be relevant to a community of other researchers, scholars, or therapists. Thus, research is not writing about one's clinical work, making up one's own theory, or sharing one's personal views.

Second, I regard this chapter as a personal narrative with some qualities of a speculative theory: I am neither researcher nor participant; I am expressing only my personal views; I am basing my ideas on my experience rather than on data; I am sharing what I know rather than seeking what I do not know; I am speculating and elaborating to some extent; and I am not offering a comprehensive theory on authenticity or integrity.

AUTHENTICITY OF PARADIGM

The second question for insuring authenticity is: Am I doing *qualitative* research? Not every research study that includes non-numerical data is conceived within a qualitative paradigm; not every researcher who claims to be a qualitative researcher has a belief system that is congruent with the paradigm. Thus, it is not the type of data or methodology used in a study that establishes the paradigm, it is the researcher's epistemological stance, i.e., the way the researcher views the nature of truth, knowledge, and knowing. Using qualitative data and methodology does not ensure that the researcher's epistemology or way of knowing and inquiring about the world is within a qualitative paradigm. Perhaps the best way to understand this is to make some comparisons between quantitative and qualitative epistemologies.

Quantitative researchers believe that absolute truth and reality exist in the form of immutable laws of nature; qualitative researchers believe that truth and reality exist in the form of multiple, intangible mental constructions. Thus, even the purpose of research is different. While quantitative researchers seek to identify or verify what is *the* truth, and to add truths together to form *valid* knowledge of reality, qualitative researchers seek to develop increasingly more viable approximations of the world.

I believe (along with many other qualitative researchers) that the basic epistemologies underlying quantitative and qualitative paradigms are mutually exclusive ways of thinking about the world, and therefore cannot be integrated or combined within the same study. I do believe that we can collect both quantitative and qualitative types of data, using both methodological approaches, and that we can do both types of research at different times, but it is logically impossible to adopt both epistemological positions regarding the nature of truth and knowledge at the same time. The basic question that a researcher seeks to answer in an inquiry is *either* positivistic in epistemology, or it is not, regardless of the types of data and methodology used. Positivistic researchers seek to establish or verify *the real* truth about something, nonpositivists examine multiple constructions of reality.

Taking all this into account, establishing the authenticity of paradigm has the following requirements: 1) being aware of how one's beliefs and values compares to the basic epistemologies of the qualitative paradigm, e.g., postpositivist, naturalist, constructivist, interpretivist, and critical theory, (Denzin and Lincoln, 1994); 2) using a methodology that fits with one's epistemology; and 3) fully disclosing any discrepancies in epistemology or methodology.

AUTHENTICITY OF FOCUS

The focus of an inquiry includes the phenomenon that the researcher has committed him/herself to study (such as a particular event or event process, an experience, an individual or group, or a material thing), and the purpose or question that the researcher has formulated with regard to it. As such, a focus is similar to what is traditionally called the "general statement of the research problem."

Authenticity of focus requires several layers of commitment and responsibility, which though they may seem rather obvious, are nevertheless of utmost significance to the integrity of the researcher and the study.

Do I Have a Focus?

First, authenticity requires that I acknowledge to myself that the study has a focus when it does and that it does not have a focus when it does not. The inauthentic stances are the following: I do not have a focus when I do, or I do have a focus when I do not. Both involve a refusal to bring the focus into awareness and then take responsibility for it in carrying out the study.

Inauthenticity at this level is most often detected in the way a researcher goes about collecting data. For example, if I am interviewing participants, I either have a focus for the study which shapes the interview or I do not. If I do have a focus, I conduct the interview using it and insure that the necessary questions are answered during the course of the interview. I then take responsibility for both the focus that I took and for the type of interview I conducted. I also sort and cull the data accordingly, that is, according to what is relevant and irrelevant to the focus.

On the other hand, if I have no focus for the study at the time of the interview, then I make no attempt to shape the interview and I take full responsibility for doing that kind of interview. I then must accept all the data equally because having no focus or question means that I have not established a priori criteria for determining the relative value, significance or relevance of the data. At this point, I have two options for responding to the data: I can either establish my own criteria for what constitutes interesting or relevant data, or I can allow trends or characteristics in the data to suggest what is most significant to me. Both options indicate that, notwithstanding my original intention to have no focus, I have now begun to focus on a certain aspect or part of the data in order establish relevance, and that I am responding to the data from a particular context or point of view.

Intentionally avoiding a focus can be very useful in establishing one and certainly this is a legitimate stance to take at certain stages of the inquiry, if fully acknowledged to both oneself and the participants. On the other hand, avoiding a focus and either admitting or excusing it smacks of inauthenticity.

Needless to say, this type of inauthenticity is particularly offensive to participants because it colors interactions and relationships in pervasive and sometimes insidious ways. The participants may feel used or manipulated to address a focus within a particular context while the researcher insists that s/he has no such focus, question or perspective.

Researchers who prefer not to establish (or acknowledge) a focus frequently espouse three values as the reason: the desire to be nondirective with participants, the goal of studying a phenomenon "holistically," and an avoidance of "reductionism."

Is Focusing Directive?

Let me say from the onset that I believe that it is impossible to be completely nondirective, whether as a therapist, a researcher, or merely as a breathing human being. To me, every interaction and communication with the world is a directive of some kind. Granted some interactions are more directive than others, but everything I do within an interaction or communication with another person impinges on or influences that person in some way. That is why we call it interaction—our two actions are intertwined. Thus, to say that I am not directing a research interview on some level is to say that I am not there. Whenever I am with others, I must take appropriate responsibility for the interaction, no matter how nondirective I hope or intend to be.

It is also important to realize that, regardless of my intention, my role in an interaction or communication can also be distorted by the other, so that even when I wish to not impinge on or influence someone, the person may perceive me as directive, and may respond as if I am. I can never be certain when I do or do not impinge on or influence the other; thus, my intention to not be directive has nothing to do with the effect I have within an interaction.

In addition to being impossible, nondirectiveness has nothing to do with having a research focus. Being nondirective is simply not the same as being unfocused, and being directive is not the same as being focused. To equate directiveness with focus is a distortion of both ways of being. This distortion may stem from a misunderstanding regarding the nature of a focus in qualitative research. To be sure, a qualitative focus is never a closed-ended, yes/no question like those posed in positivistic research; it is much more open-ended. But here again, open-ended does not mean unfocused. If I ask you to describe a particular experience, such as participating in a group drum improvisation that I know you have experienced, I am focusing your attention on a particular topic, I am defining what is relevant to the immediate research discussion, but I am not intentionally limiting or directing your answer—you can say whatever you wish about the experience.

If my study has a much more specific focus, let us say, physical reactions to the drum improvisation, I can proceed with the same clarity, however now I only know that you have had the experience of improvising on the drum; I cannot assume that your experience included physical reactions. Thus, I may begin by asking you to describe your experience of improvising, and then if you do not mention physical reactions, ask whether your experience involved them. How else will you ever know the real question I am asking if I do not ask it? It is inauthentic to say that the focus of my study is physical reactions, and then wait to see whether you ever bring them up on your own. If you spontaneously bring up physical reactions without my asking, can I really conclude that you thought they were the most relevant dimensions of the experience to tell me? And if you do not mention them without my asking, can I infer that they were not relevant dimensions? Open-ended questions, like closed-ended questions, can be focused or unfocused, directive or nondirective, and clear or unclear.

There is only one way out of this dilemma: if I have a focus, I acknowledge the focus whether trying to be directive or nondirective, and I am authentic about it when gathering data. Authenticity is not a form of control, it is a way of relating clearly to myself and to others.

Is Focusing Holistic?

As for holism, the same two arguments apply. First, like nondirectiveness, being holistic is an ideal that is impossible to ever fully meet. Human beings simply do not have the power to grasp or completely know the whole of anyone or anything. Certainly we can strive to conceive of persons and phenomena in their wholeness and as comprehensively as possible (which is how I define holism), but as soon as we presume success, that we have in fact captured everything about the whole in its entirety, we run the risk of inauthenticity.

The second argument is that even if it were possible, being holistic has nothing to do with being focused, the two cannot be equated. When I am striving to be holistic, I may be focused or unfocused; and when I am not striving to be holistic, I may be focused or unfocused.

For the sake of example, let us suppose that I am observing the drum improvisation session. When I try to include *everything* about the session in my observation, sooner or later I must confront the delusion. I simply cannot take in everything that is there to see, hear, sense and know; there is too much. There are musical events, nonmusical events, physical reactions and emotional reactions, interactions between participants, the meaning given to the music and the experience, and all those things that are out of our awareness about the phenomenon itself. The possibilities for awareness are inexhaustible. To be authentic, I must acknowledge that, as much as I try, it is impossible to be *completely* holistic.

Taking this issue from another perspective, to be authentic, I must also acknowledge the impossibility of *not* focusing, even when I am trying to be holistic. If I conduct the observation through a videotape, I am already focusing on the visual event sequence and I either take responsibility for favoring the visual field or I do not. I either take responsibility for focusing the study on events rather than experiences or I do not. Moreover, within the visual field, the lens of the camera becomes an even narrower focus and I either accept responsibility for directing the lens or I do not. And even staying within the lens, I can choose to focus on the client, the therapist, the interactions, the music, their movements, their words, their experiences, and so forth. Again, I either take responsibility for focusing on one and not another, or I do not.

To be holistic does not require me to have no focus; and to have no focus does not make me holistic. To believe so is illogical and ultimately leads to inauthenticity.

Is Focusing Reductionistic?

A related confusion is equating focusing with reductionism, a practice in quantitative research (which is copiously avoided in qualitative research) wherein the phenomenon under study is defined "operationally," that is, only in terms of variables which can be accurately observed and measured. The phenomenon is considered to be "reduced" because the whole of it is defined only in terms of a quantifiable part of it, that is, the variable(s) which can be measured. Thus, for example, short-term memory becomes defined as the number of digits that can be immediately recalled, intelligence becomes defined as the composite score on a test, and so forth.

In contrast, qualitative researchers seek to study all discernible facets of a phenomenon, while also avoiding reduction of the phenomenon to any one of its facets. In this regard, qualitative researchers *do* in fact strive to be holistic (as defined and delimited above).

Here again, focusing has nothing to do with reducing a whole to any of its parts. Rather, to focus is to define what the boundaries of the whole are for research purposes. It is the difference between operationally defining melodic creativity as the number of new motifs generated in an improvisation, and focusing an improvisation inquiry on melodic creativity in all of its ramifications. To reduce is to replace the whole phenomenon with a quantifiable part of it, to focus is to define what is regarded the whole of the phenomenon for purposes of research.

Is the Focus Mine?

To be authentic, a researcher has to take full responsibility for selecting the focus. That is, the focus of a research study should always belong to the researcher, not to anyone else. Key questions are: Precisely whose study am I doing, mine or someone else's? If I am doing someone else's, do I accept the focus?

Inauthentic stances occur when I believe that someone else has given the study its focus rather than acknowledging that I formulated or accepted it; or when I claim authorship of the focus when it does in fact belong to someone else. This threat to authenticity occurs most often with students doing master's theses or doctoral dissertation research who work under supervision by their professors, or professional researchers who work for an agency that has specific research agendas.

Another related inauthentic stance is when I claim that the data revealed the focus to me so that the focus came from the data rather than from what I brought to the data in order to recognize what the data revealed.

Is the Focus the Focus?

Authenticity requires that the focus of the study *is* the focus—that I *am* studying whom and what I think I am studying. There should be no discrepancy between what I think is my focus and the data that I am gathering.

In the qualitative paradigm, much attention is given to the multilayered nature of reality and the many different constructions of reality that are possible. Authenticity of focus requires that the researcher be aware of which layers and constructions are of prime interest in the inquiry.

To continue with the example of an improvisation study, I have several options in establishing the focus. I can focus on various aspects of what occurred:

In-vivo events and interactions. These can take place during a particular improvisation or session and be examined through live and videotaped observations. The focus may be further specified with regard to the kinds of events of interest, e.g., musical, verbal, and/or nonverbal events and interactions, and the specific individuals of interest (the client, the therapist, client-client interactions, client-therapist interactions, etc.).

The actual improvisation itself. This exists as analyzed musically by the therapist and/or researcher. Here the focus is not on the events or experiences but on the musical material itself.

How the client and/or therapist experienced the events, interactions or musical improvisation. This can be gleaned from their verbal reports within the session itself. Here the aim is to obtain a basic description of the content and nature of the experience itself, e.g., what happened, what was perceived or noticed, sensations and feelings, thoughts during the improvisation. The focus may be further delimited to a particular experience or class of experiences, e.g., playing the drum, times during which the improvisers felt they were in harmony with one another.

How the client and/or therapist construed the events, interactions or music. That is, what meaning or significance they gave to the experience as gleaned from an interview after a short time lapse. Note that the previous layer is immediate and involves mere description of the experience whereas this one involves time lapse and some form of analysis or interpretation of the experience.

How the client and/or therapist reconstruct the experience. This would occur after having a longer time lapse and other similar experiences with improvisation. This layer can be examined through re-creations of the original improvisation, re-experiencing the improvisation by listening or viewing a tape of it, reminiscing through the experience imaginally, etc. Here, time and other experiences have probably given the experiencer a broader and more historical perspective on the original experience, so that the meaning and significance of it may be different from the previous layer.

The client or therapist as an individual. This can be examined through any or all of the previous layers, and through observations and/or interviews. Here the focus is on the person as improviser rather than on the improvisation or his/her experiences, constructions and reconstructions of it.

Constructions and reconstructions of the researcher. Here the focus shifts from the constructions or reconstructions of the actual parties involved in the improvisation to a third party, the researcher or observer. At this layer then, the researcher constructs and reconstructs the events, interactions, music, experiences as reported by the client and/or therapist, and/or the constructions and reconstructions already given by the client and/or therapist.

Authenticity of focus requires that the researcher be aware of exactly what s/he is studying. If I focus on events and interactions, then I must acknowledge that I am not focusing on the music per se or the improviser's experiences of it, and I must also decide whose constructions and reconstructions I will be examining, mine as researcher or theirs as client or therapist.

Inauthenticity creeps in very easily here. For example, I can think that my focus is on what they did, but I may actually be studying what I think they did, or only their experience of what they did; I can think that my focus is on their music, but I may be examining only my visual observations of the events and interactions surrounding the music. And of course, there is always the danger of the "holistic" inauthenticity: I am focusing on all of these things.

IS THE PURPOSE THE PURPOSE?

People are motivated to do research for many different reasons, personal, professional, social, political and otherwise. Authenticity requires that researchers be aware of their own motives, so that the stated purpose of the study is in fact the purpose, and the beneficiaries of the study are in fact the beneficiaries. Here are some possibilities:

> I am studying him so he can understand himself.
> I am studying him so I can understand him.
> I am studying him so I can understand therapy.
> I am studying him so you can understand him.
> I am studying him so you can understand me.
> I am studying me so I can understand him.
> I am studying me so I can understand me.
> I am studying him and me so I/he/you can understand us.
> I am studying music therapy so I/you/he can understand him.
> I am studying music therapy so I/you/he can understand it.
> I am studying music therapy so I/you/he can understand me.

Of course, we can also take this one step further, by adding onto the above statements hidden agendas and personal motives:

> . . . so that I can prove myself to me.
> . . . so that I can prove myself to you.
> . . . so that I can prove you right or wrong.
> . . . so that I can prove music therapy works.
> . . . so that I can gain your recognition or approval.
> . . . so that you recognize the importance of music therapy.

Not much more needs to be said about this kind of inauthenticity as it is usually easy to detect in both self and others. What needs to be kept in mind is that the stated purpose of the study should be a purpose that is directly related to the focus and the participants; it should not be contaminated by any hidden agendas or personal motives of the researcher.

AUTHENTICITY OF CONTEXT

The context of an inquiry includes all those personal, professional, interpersonal, and environmental factors or conditions that may be operating and affecting the research process. These factors and conditions may influence the focus or purpose of the study, the way the researcher interacts with participants and colleagues, the way the data are gathered and analyzed, and the way the findings are communicated.

To be authentic is to continually bring these myriad contexts into awareness and to take responsibility for them as appropriate. Several contexts require special attention with regard to authenticity: the personal context of the researcher, the professional stance of the researcher, and the interpersonal environment. Put together, these contexts constitute "where I am coming from" as researcher.

Who Am I as a Person?

Who I am as a person provides a context for everything I do as a researcher. When I engage in the inquiry process, I bring to it my personality, my body, my conscious and unconscious motivations, my constructs about life, my emotional needs, my spiritual beliefs, and a particular style of understanding and relating to the world, all of which play an integral part in how I go about setting and accomplishing my research objectives. What I am proposing here is that, like therapists, researchers also have "countertransference" issues which directly affect their work, and researchers also have to make continual efforts to bring them into awareness, to channel or manage them as indicated.

I hasten to add two qualifying comments. First, I am not suggesting that researchers go into therapy whenever undertaking a project. Rather I believe they should enter into a self-inquiry process that helps them to examine their own personal attitudes at each stage of the research process. More will be said of this later.

Second, I would like to clarify the level of awareness that I feel is necessary and sufficient for a researcher to channel or manage such personal matters. I believe that there are several levels of consciousness within any countertransference—whether operating in therapy or research—and that only certain levels are accessible, depending on their content: 1) some things about myself are already in my consciousness, and at various stages of being integrated into it; 2) some things may be in the process of entering into my consciousness, but still require some effort on my part before fully integrating into it; 3) some things are available to my consciousness, but will not enter into or integrate into my consciousness unless I have some kind of assistance from another person; and, 4) some things are unavailable to my consciousness, lying stubbornly within my unconscious regardless of any intervention by myself or others. All I can do as a researcher is to work with the upper three levels. By definition the last level is unconscious and therefore inaccessible, at least for a particular time period.

Given human nature to keep out of consciousness anything which is difficult to accept or integrate into it, and given the pervasive influence that the personal context can have, authenticity requires an ongoing process of self-inquiry. The primary focus is to determine how personal needs or issues may be influencing each stage or step within the research process. Important questions include the following:

* Is the focus and purpose of the study related in any way to questions and goals that I struggle with in my own life?

* For whom am I answering this question, in addition to the intended research audience? Does my commitment to the focus and purpose of the study resemble the way I commit myself to other things in my personal life?

* Does my decision-making as a researcher resemble the way I make life decisions?

* When gathering data, am I interacting with the persons involved in the research in ways that resemble how I relate (or need to relate) to persons in my life?

* When making sense of the data, am I encountering the same strengths and obstacles as I do when I try to make sense of my life? Do the same things bother and baffle me? Do I make the same assumptions and distortions?

* When I communicate the findings of my research, do I encounter the same communication problems found in my relationships?

* How does each aspect or phase of the study make me feel?

Inauthenticity usually occurs when the researcher fails to acknowledge or take responsibility for where s/he is coming from personally and how this is affecting the study. Typical inauthentic stances include these perspectives: Who I am has nothing to do with what I am doing as a researcher. I think I am aware of my personal context and its influence (when I am not). I have no power to monitor the effects of who I am on the researcher (when I do).

Who Am I as a Professional?

The difference between personal and professional contexts is that the former is concerned with the self, thus constituting the personal baggage that I bring to the research and the latter is concerned with the research itself, thus constituting the professional baggage that I carry along. Professional baggage includes my opinions and biases regarding the field of study, my philosophy regarding research, my competence as a researcher, my theoretical orientation regarding the topic, the constructs I have already formed with regard to the focus, purpose, and data in the study, and all the assumptions that I make about the content and structure of my research study.

Qualitative researchers have different opinions on whether such professional biases and stances can and should be bracketed or controlled in some way. Some believe that it is impossible, some believe it is undesirable, and some believe that it is both possible and desirable. Thus, one's opinion on this is itself a stance.

To be authentic here requires that I continually seek to uncover what my professional stances and assumptions are and take full responsibility for either using, ignoring, or bracketing them. The best way to do this is to consult frequently with colleagues, including those who have different as well as similar viewpoints.

Typical inauthentic stances are: My professional biases have not influenced the research process (when they have); and I have the power to bracket my professional biases (when I do not).

Who Am I as a Researcher?

Research involves multifaceted interactions and relationships with participants, agencies, other therapists, co-researchers, consultants and readers. Authenticity requires that I remain aware of and take appropriate responsibility for the nature of these relationships and my roles within them. For example, when I am researcher, I relate to the participants in the role of researcher, and take appropriate responsibility for the nature of this relationship; as researcher, I strive to be aware of the interpersonal dynamics involved in gathering data, and take appropriate responsibility for the kinds of interactions that take place.

Because the qualitative paradigm is predicated on the importance of understanding the reciprocal relationship between observer and observed, or researcher and participant, it is very important for the researcher to understand the study (its focus, purpose, data gathering procedures) from the participant's point of view. The empathy and intersubjectivity that a researcher must develop, however, has to be authentic; it is not enough that I assume I know how it feels to be a participant in the study, or that I assume that I understand the participant from his/her point of view. I therefore recommend that, whenever possible, all researchers be a participant in their own study or experience whatever the participants experience. These data may or may not be included in the study; most importantly, they should be taken into account when analyzing and interpreting data from the participants.

AUTHENTICITY OF METHOD

Are There Rules?

Authenticity of method requires that I acknowledge the freedom that I have to choose the ways in which I gather and process data, and take responsibility for that freedom. Unlike quantitative research—where specific, predetermined and replicable methods must be used appropriately in order to insure the integrity of the research—qualitative researchers can create new methods for each situation as the need arises and with very few expectations for replicability. Although this may sound as if quantitative research has lots of rules and qualitative research does not, this is not at all the case; in fact, inauthenticity of method stems from an assumption that either there are no rules in qualitative research when there are, or conversely, that there are rules when there are not.

To say that qualitative researchers design their own methods is not to say that they are free to do anything that strikes their fancy, and that this will not affect the integrity of the study. There are a few rules, and these rules are aimed at integrity issues! The first and cardinal rule is that the method a researcher uses to accomplish the purpose of the study must be responsive to and appropriate for the phenomenon and participants under investigation. Put another way, integrity requires that the researcher be free to use any method that s/he feels can best accommodate the phenomenon and participants while also accomplishing the purposes of the study.

This rule can be applied inauthentically in two ways. The first is to deny that it is a rule, and to assume that, as a qualitative researcher, I can do whatever I want. This is an example of believing that there are no rules when there are, or at the extreme, that no rule is the rule. This inauthentic stance is most often taken by professionals who like to take the "high ground" and be forever above or ahead of their colleagues, and thus beyond or exempt from all rules—they can be authentic, and scholarly, and creative researchers by doing whatever they do. I notice that this kind of inauthenticity is usually linked to a confusion of boundaries between what constitutes research and what does not. For these high-minded (and sometimes narcissistic) professionals, everything they do is everything—that is, everything they do is research, everything they do is creativity, and so forth. Also, for them, theory is equated with research, research is the same as clinical work, clinical work is music-making, and music-making is research. Notice that this inauthenticity is closely related to a distortion of intent and paradigm, as discussed earlier.

The second inauthenticity is that this rule (to match the method with the phenomenon and participants) takes away my freedom to choose appropriate methods. Here, instead of taking responsibility for designing, choosing, or applying a method, I assert that the method was determined solely by the phenomenon and participants. Essentially, I refuse to own the personal choices and professional judgments that I have made.

The third inauthenticity is that there is a rule that determines what method I should use, when there is not. Here the researcher tries to justify the method s/he used by asserting that its part of the paradigm. A good example is when a researcher believes that every interview must be open-ended and nondirective, when this is not a rule. The rule is that when the phenomenon and participants call for this kind of interview I do it, and when they do not, I may not, depending upon what the focus of the study is. In short, the paradigm does not make me do anything!

When this rule of appropriate methodology is applied authentically, researchers quickly discover a second rule: that methods of qualitative research are shaped through reciprocal interactions between the phenomenon, participants, and researcher, with each having equal power and responsibility over its shaping. It is therefore inauthentic to assert that the method was determined by the phenomenon when it was not, or to claim that the method was dictated by the participants when it was not. Authenticity requires that I look at how all these forces have interacted to shape the method, and to take responsibility for which forces played a greater role.

AUTHENTICITY OF FINDINGS

Am I Open to Discovery?

As I begin to gather and process data, I do so with expectations and hopes—some more conscious than others, and some more important than others—so that by the time the findings begin to emerge, I have already developed a stance in relation to them. In plain words, I either expected the results that I got or I did not and I either wanted them or I did not. It is natural to have these expectations and hopes, and in fact it is unusual for a researcher not to have a vested interest in the findings of a study.

Authenticity requires that I be aware of and acknowledge these expectations and hopes and take responsibility for them when processing the data. Essentially, I have to be receptive to discovering whatever is there while also ensuring that my expectations and hopes are neither filtering out what is there or fabricating what is not there. As a researcher, I must remain fully open to discovering whatever the data reveals, whether it be expected or unexpected, wanted or unwanted.

To be fully open to the findings also means that I will recognize those that are not already in my awareness. As researcher, I will welcome new, unexpected, unsolicited and serendipitous findings. I do not have to already know what I sought to discover; I can be surprised. On the other hand, I must also be open to those findings that were already in my awareness.

To be fully open to the findings means that I will recognize findings that are unflattering to me. This includes those that are contradictory to my thinking or previous research, or discoveries that point out my shortcomings as a therapist or researcher. I must accept both contradicting and unflattering findings, and I must be wary of findings that either flatter me or shift the responsibility for errors or inadequacies away from me. On the other hand, I must also be open to findings that put me in a good light.

Finally, to be fully open means that I can recognize and acknowledge discoveries that are not my own. I do not have to be the discoverer of most of the important findings; participants and others involved in the study may also make important discoveries. On the other hand, I must acknowledge those findings that are mine as mine.

AUTHENTICITY OF COMMUNICATION

No matter how earnestly we try, we can never tell the whole story of our research. A research report is at best a skeletal communication of the vast array of experiences and discoveries that took place during the inquiry process.

Authenticity of communication first requires that I acknowledge that I can only tell you part of the story, and that it is not within my power to tell you everything. With this comes a freedom to choose what I will and will not communicate to my readers, and a need to take responsibility for that choice.

There are no rules for what *must* be included in *every* qualitative research report—only I as researcher determine what will be in the report and what will not. On the other hand, to say that there are no codes or standards for communication is also fallacious. Here again we have the danger of taking the position that there are certain rules (that I must obey) when there are no such rules, or that there are no rules (that I must obey) when there are. Ultimately, I will be unable to hide in either position.

The primary dilemma in being an authentic communicator is that as a researcher I do not want you, the reader, to know something about me that is either too disparaging or intimate, and yet if I tell you what you should know about the study, you will probably discover them. Thus, a major risk of authentic communication is unwanted self-disclosures.

There are at least three inauthentic ways out of this dilemma. In the first, I can present to you who I am not, or not present to you who I am. Here I communicate behind a mask and manage your impressions of me. Of course, the inauthenticity here is believing that I have the power to fully manage your impressions of me when I do not and that I have the power to hide myself when I do not.

In the second, I can avoid taking responsibility for what I am communicating. Rather than take and claim my own voice when making "I" statements, I instead project my voice through other persons, such as the participants, colleagues, or readers. This stance is communication without clarity of boundaries and self-responsibility. To be authentic, I cannot say what I want to say or what needs to be said and then equate my voice with those of anyone else; nor can I take their voices as mine when communicating what they said. I can only have one voice, and it is mine and only mine; it is not anyone else's and theirs is not mine.

Finally, I can withhold information about the study that is too self-disclosing. This stance is deception by omission. It is like the mask option except that instead of hiding myself I hide things about the research study. To be authentic requires that I acknowledge to the reader that, due to its personal nature, I am omitting something from the report.

In summary, authenticity of communication mandates a few requirements: first, that I communicate who I am as accurately as I can, while also acknowledging the limits of my own self-consciousness; second, that I communicate whatever I believe is necessary for the reader to know in order to fully engage the data and findings as I have; and third, that I take appropriate responsibility for what I choose to communicate while also acknowledging that I cannot communicate everything or through anyone else.

SUMMARY

Authenticity is being who I am. It is an at-oneness between consciousness, intention, experience, and action. As a researcher, authenticity is manifested in the kind of research I do, how I focus my efforts, the way I collect and process data, the discoveries I make, and how I communicate them. During these stages of inquiry there are several authenticity statements that a researcher should try on to determine how well they fit:

* I am doing research.

* I am operating within a qualitative point of view.

* My methods are consistent with my point of view.

* I do (or do not) have a focus.

* Having a focus allows me to be either directive or nondirective, holistic or nonholistic.

* The focus is my focus, not anyone else's.

* The focus is as I have formulated it.

* The purpose is as I have stated it, apart from any other agendas or motives.

* I am aware of and take responsibility for the personal context in which I conducted this research.

* I am aware of and take responsibility for the professional stances I have brought to this research.

* I am aware of and take responsibility for the roles and relationships I have had while conducting this inquiry.

* I am open to using a methodology that evolves from my mutual interactions with the phenomenon, participants, and paradigm.

* I take appropriate responsibility for the methodological rules and procedures I have chosen to apply in gathering and processing the data.

* I am open to making discoveries that are expected and unexpected, wanted and unwanted, in my awareness and out of my awareness, flattering and unflattering, contradictory and consistent.

* I have accurately communicated who I am.

* I take responsibility for what I have and have not communicated.

* I have communicated what I believe is essential for the reader to know to engage the data and findings as I have.

In closing, I would like to quote something that Dag Hammersjold said in a different context, but which relates very directly to the challenge of being authentic as a researcher, and especially in music therapy:

> The more faithfully you listen to the voice within you, the better you will hear what is sounding outside. (Gardner & Reese, 1975, p. 122)

REFERENCES

Denzin, N., & Lincoln, Y. (Eds.). (1994). *Handbook of qualitative research*. Newbury Park, CA: Sage Publications.

Gardner, J., Reese, F. (1975). *Quotations of wit and wisdom*. New York: W. W. Norton.

Guba, E., & Lincoln, Y. (1989). *Fourth generation evaluation*. Newbury Park, CA: Sage.

Lincoln, Y., & Guba, E. (1985). *Naturalistic inquiry*. Newbury Park, CA: Sage Publications.

Moustakas, C. (1990). *Heuristic research: Design, methodology and applications*. Newbury Park, CA: Sage Publications.

Experiencing Music Therapy: Meaningful Moments in the Music Therapy Process

Dorit Amir

INTRODUCTION

In this paper I want to talk about a qualitative research project I undertook as my doctoral dissertation (Amir, 1992). Let me begin by telling you a story about a girl named Shir. Shir was four-years-old when she was referred to me by her psychologist for music therapy sessions. The reason for referral was elective mutism. The only place Shir spoke was at home with her parents and her dolls. She did not speak outside of her home; she was mute. Shir went to kindergarten and participated in all indoor activities, but she did not talk.

When she first came in, I saw a beautiful little girl who clung to her mother and would not come into the music therapy room. I took the autoharp out of my room to the hallway and strummed it very softly. Shir let go of her mother's hand and hesitantly followed me into the room. I went to the far corner of the small room playing the autoharp while she stood next to the door looking down to the floor. Occasionally, she would lift her head up and make eye contact with me for a few seconds. She looked very sad and I still remember how every time she would make eye contact I would feel a moment of connection with her.

During her third session, she sat next to the door, as usual, looking at the autoharp which was on my lap in a far corner of the room. I improvised on the autoharp and she started crawling toward me until she finally sat next to my lap. Something within me told me to stop playing. After a few seconds of silence, she put her hand on the autoharp and strummed it once. She looked at me and smiled; I smiled, too. What a precious moment it was.

In the sessions that followed, she became more active and discovered the drum, experimenting with it. It was during her tenth session that she started beating the drum, softly and slowly, gradually increasing the tempo and volume. The sound grew louder and faster. She was using both hands and it looked like she was fully involved. The drumming became very intense until it reached a peak. Shir screamed, started to cry, and came to me. Automatically, I opened my arms, hugged her, and held her very close. This was a very intimate moment for me. The beauty of this moment moved me.

This is one example of many special moments that occurred during my work as a music therapist. These particular moments stood out for me as they occurred. They are still riveting for me to recall. While trying to find words that can describe what was happening during these moments I was struck by the number of descriptors that popped into my mind: beauty, love, intuition, insight, peak experience, intimacy, spiritual, Aha!, transpersonal, transcendent, aesthetic, creativity, flow of energy, contact, healing, transformation, change, growth, expansion, turning point, breakthrough, inspiration, catharsis, spontaneity, immediacy, liberation, openness, oneness . . .

The motivation for doing the research and the decision for a topic came directly from my own clinical experience and personal interest in these experiences. I wanted to find out more about the meaning of the experience of music therapy for those who are involved as therapists and clients.

RESEARCH QUESTIONS

The basic question of the study was: How can we describe and under-stand the experience of music therapy—including the complexities of subjective realities and multilevel intrapersonal relationships and relationships between client(s) and music therapist(s)—in an authentic manner?

Additionally, I sought insight into the following questions:

1) What are the meaningful moments in the music therapy process as perceived by music therapists?

2) How do music therapists describe their experience during these moments?

3) What is the importance of these moments to music therapists?

4) What are the meaningful moments in the music therapy process as perceived by music therapy clients?

5) How do clients describe their experience during these moments?

6) What is the importance of these moments to clients?

7) What are the contributing factors?

8) How do the perceptions and descriptions of these moments compare between therapists and clients?

METHOD

Introduction and Rationale

In order to illuminate how meaningful moments in the music therapy process were experienced by both therapists and clients, a qualitative method of data gathering and analysis was used to establish a grounded theory (Glaser & Strauss, 1967).

Grounded theory entails the creation of theory by systematically and intensively analyzing the data—often sentence by sentence or phrase by phrase—contained in field notes, interviews, or other documents. These are analyzed by constant comparison, data are extensively collected and coded, thus producing a well constructed theory. The focus of analysis is not merely collecting or ordering a mass of data, but on organizing many ideas which have emerged from analysis of the data (Glaser & Strauss, 1967).

The search for grounded theory leads to the generation of new theory based on comprehensive description, analysis and interpretation of data.

Research Participants

The criteria for music therapists who could be participants in this research were those music therapists who, at the time of the project, had the following characteristics:

1) Doing psychotherapeutically oriented work from a humanistic perspective, i.e., those who saw the goal of music therapy as helping clients to get in touch with the creative self and move toward emotional health and self-fulfillment.

2) Held an M.A. degree in music therapy and were certified or registered music therapists at the time of the research project.

3) Practicing clinicians with at least five years of experience.

These criteria were not meant to imply that meaningful moments do not occur in other approaches to music therapy, or that other candidates with less experience could not have been chosen for this kind of a study. Qualitative inquiry, however, uses *purposive sampling*. Purposive sampling enabled me to choose participants who appeared most likely to serve as the best informants for this particular study, thus maximizing the possibility that a fuller picture of multiple realities would be uncovered.

The criteria for clients were:

1) At least four months of ongoing group or individual music therapy.

2) Verbal abilities sufficient to be able to describe their experiences in a rich and full manner.

All together, I had eight participants: four music therapists and four clients. Three clients were in private music therapy and one was receiving music therapy in a rehabilitation center.

After conducting second interviews with six of the participants, gathering the data and analyzing all the interviews, the data started to repeat. Additional data and analysis no longer contributed to the discovery of new categories. According to Margo Ely et al. (1991), "the analysis ends when new data no longer generate new insights" (p. 177). Thus, I stayed with eight participants in the study: four music therapists and four music therapy clients. Lofland & Lofland (1984) encourage researchers to work with a small number of participants: "A small sample allows the researcher to develop 'intimate familiarity' with the participants. It enables the researcher to obtain the rich, detailed materials that can be used in qualitative analysis" (p. 11-12).

Research Instrument: The Intensive Interview

Because the experience of a music therapist involves internal aspects that cannot be easily observed, I utilized in-depth interviewing as a method of data collection. In general, I used Spradley's (1979) concept of the ethnographic interview as a guide in conducting the interviews. An ethnographic interview is "a series of friendly conversations into which the researcher slowly introduces new elements to assist informants to respond as informants" (p. 58).

All interviews consisted of open-ended, descriptive questions. Because of its nature, the interviewer's focus in this kind of interview was on what the participants had to say about their experience. Therefore, it was possible to have only a beginning set of questions. All of the interviews started with the same question: When you think about your experience as a music therapist (or as a client in music therapy) what comes to your mind?

Data Analysis

Qualitative data analysis is a thorough examination of data in an effort to establish meaning. "The product of analysis is a creation that speaks to the heart of what was learned" (Ely et al., 1991, p. 140).

It is important to say that the analysis of data is a process that begins with the first interview and goes hand in hand with the gathering of data.

The basic operation of qualitative analysis is the following: First comes the collection of data consisting of interview protocols and the researcher's observer comments, process notes and analytic memos (Bogdan & Biklen, 1982; Ely et al., 1991; Strauss, 1987). Next is the creation of thinking units that can be useful in organizing and categorizing the data (Bogdan & Biklen, 1982; Ely et al., 1991). This is followed by the establishment of a set of categories that arise from the data. "Creating categories, subcategories and discovering their links brings a researcher into intimate reacquaintance with the data" (Ely et al., 1991, p. 145). What follows is the discovery of a core category which is related to as many categories and subcategories as possible and "is central to the integration of the findings" (Strauss, 1987, p. 21). Then comes the unifying, re-shaping and re-organizing of categories. "The original list of categories will be reducible in size because of improved articulation and integration. At the same time the categories become saturated, that is, so well defined that there is no point in adding further exemplars to them" (Lincoln & Guba, 1981, pp. 343-344). Last is writing the theory, where identification of themes, topics and patterns that characterize the phenomenon under study is provided in a clear and comprehensive format.

Data Analysis in this Study. This basic operation served as a framework for my analysis which consisted of nine stages:

1.1 All interviews were audiotaped and transcribed verbatim.
1.2 I added comments about my own feelings, thoughts and impressions throughout the interview.

2.1 I started to become familiar with the content of each interview through listening to the tapes and reading the transcribed material.
2.2 I created an initial organization of data into categories for each interview. For example:

> client's\therapist's background information;
> client's\therapist's examples of meaningful moments;
> client's\therapist's feelings, images, reactions, and explanations about the meaning of the experience for them.

3.1 I read the transcriptions and listened to each interview for a second time.
3.2 I came up with further lists of categories, such as: client's\therapist's emotional reactions, physical reactions, and spiritual feelings and meanings; description of the music; description of the context.

4.1 I re-read each transcription and the analysis of each interview.
4.2 I started to refine the categories by finding core and sub-categories for each interview. This was done by cross-analysis of the different examples in each interview. For example: client's\therapist's intrapersonal experience; client's\therapist's emotional, physical, spiritual reactions.

4.3 New core categories were discovered. For example:

> conditions that allowed client\therapist to have these intrapersonal experiences;
> client's\therapist's perception of themselves;
> client's readiness and commitment;
> client's\therapist's perception of music and music therapy trust;
> client-therapist relationship.

5.1 At this point I wrote profiles for each participant. The profiles included three main parts:
   A. basic information about the participant;
   B. description and analysis of each example of participant's meaningful experience;
   C. a cross-analysis of all examples, which included three core categories:

   i. components and characteristics of all examples
   ii. conditions that spawned these experiences
   iii. contribution of these experiences to participants' lives.

6.1 This step included a second level analysis: cross-analysis of all four clients' profiles and all four therapists' profiles.
6.2 I compared the three core categories of the cross-analysis in each profile and organized them. For example: all the clients' intrapersonal experiences were put together and became a core category while each component and characteristic of these experiences became sub-categories.

Clients' Intrapersonal Experiences

A sense of freedom
A sense of spirituality
A sense of intimacy
Insight
A sense of integration
A sense of being whole

The same was done with the other two core categories: conditions and contributions.

7.1   At this time I had two sets of analyses: one pertaining to clients' profiles, and the other including therapists' profiles. I re-read what I did in step five and started to see that each component was, in fact, a meaningful moment in the process of music therapy, as described by clients and therapists. So, the sub-categories changed to moments of insight, moments of freedom, moments of spirituality, and moments of intimacy.

7.2   I compared moments that emerged in the clients' cross-analysis with moments of the music therapists' cross-analysis and saw that out of fifteen moments, twelve were the same.

8.1   I organized all the moments, conditions and contributions of these moments of both clients and therapists and further refined the categories. For example: in the clients' analysis I had moments of accomplishment. The music therapists talked about their clients' moments of achievement and their own moments of feeling proud and good after their clients had a strong moment. It became clear that all three could be organized under the same category: moments of completion and accomplishment.

9.1   At this final stage I organized the findings in two sections:

  A.   The first section consisted of eight profiles: four clients and four music therapists. Each profile included background information about the participant and two to three vignettes consisting of the participants' verbatim descriptions. Ely et al. (1991) describe the function of a vignette: "The intention is to present in miniature the essence of what the researcher has seen and heard" (p. 154).

  B.   The second section consisted of the second level analysis which stemmed from the previous step.

Trustworthiness of the Study

The following are the procedures I followed to ensure trustworthiness:

Intensive contact with the participants and the phenomenon under study. With all the participants I conducted intensive interviews until I felt that no additional material surfaced in spite of probing. I feel that I achieved a close contact with the phenomenon under study through my becoming thoroughly familiar with the content of the interviews. I did this by repeated listening to the tapes and reading the transcriptions and the process notes.

Triangulation. This is a cross checking of "specific data items of a factual nature" (Lincoln & Guba, 1989, p. 241). Part of the cross checking was done during the first interview where I asked the participants to clarify certain concepts that they used.

Peer debriefing. This "is a process of exposing oneself to a peer in a manner paralleling an analytic session and for the purpose of exploring aspects of the inquiry that might otherwise remain only implicit within the inquirer's mind" (Lincoln & Guba, 1989, p. 308). Throughout the study, I participated in a peer support group consisting of three doctoral students engaged in qualitative studies. I reported and shared with the group some of the interviews and all of my analysis throughout the process. The group members assisted me in developing and checking categories and emerging theory and gave me support and nurturing whenever I needed it. At the same time, I gave other profiles to two of my music therapy colleagues in order to get their opinions, which helped me to re-shape and refine my theory.

Negative case analysis. Findings that disconfirmed categories, patterns, and themes were searched and analyzed. Categories were consistently re-defined until I resolved most of the negative cases. One negative case that was significant was included in the findings and appears under "No improvement outside therapy."

Member checks. This is a process "whereby data, analytic categories, interpretations and conclusions are tested with members of those stakeholding groups from whom the data were originally collected" (Lincoln & Guba, 1989, p. 314). While conducting second interviews with my participants, I checked some of the findings with each of them. When the profiles were ready, I gave six participants their personal profiles, and asked them to check the categories against their own experience. This was done in order to ensure that I understood meanings as participants intended to convey them. A few of the participants corrected some of the findings and these corrections were included in the final analysis.

FINDINGS

Throughout my analysis, I found fifteen distinct elements that comprised the experiences of music therapists and clients in music therapy. All of these experiences occurred in time: they took place in the beginning, middle, or end of a music therapy session. Most of them occurred in the middle and toward the end of the process that lasted from a few days to several years. As a result, all fifteen elements took place in real time. They lasted from two seconds to a few minutes within the session.

In addition, I found that these elements were experienced in a different sense of time that had nothing to do with concrete time. Statements such as the following appeared throughout the interviews: "I wasn't aware of how much time had passed;" "I couldn't believe that time had passed so quickly;" and, "It took only two seconds but my experience was that it took much longer than that because so much was happening inside me." These statements show that even though the elements occurred in real time, they were experienced in an inner, different experience of time. All participants described themselves as being lost in their experience.

I decided to call these elements "moments." According to Webster's dictionary, (1985), the word "moment" means a point in time which has a tendency to produce motion.

The Context of These Moments

All meaningful moments occurred within the context of music therapy. There were individual music therapy sessions that took place in the music therapist's home or office with Kathy, Karen and Lyn as clients and Adam and Lucy as therapists. There were individual and group music therapy sessions as a service being offered in a clinical setting. These included Ben as client, Martha, Adam and Beth as therapists. There was group music therapy that was being offered as a part of a music therapy training program (Kathy), and group music therapy that was being offered as a five-day intensive program (Lucy).

Most meaningful moments for clients and music therapists occurred while playing music. The rest occurred during discussions in the session, during other creative activities in the session and during my interviews.

Live and recorded music was used in these sessions. The live music took different forms: vocal and instrumental improvisation, singing classical and Yiddish folk songs, composing and singing one's own songs, singing gospel songs and rapping, and improvised songs. Beth used her voice, piano, guitar and various rhythm instruments with her clients. Martha used her voice and the accordion with her patients. Lucy used her voice and piano and Adam played piano, guitar, bass and sang. Several of the moments included some kind of body work and breathing in addition to the music (Lucy and Adam). Ben sang, improvised, and composed his own songs with the help of his music therapist who played the guitar. Kathy's moments contained vocal improvisations that were created by her with the musical support of her therapist with voice and/or piano, and group instrumental improvisation. Lyn's moments contained live musical improvisation, mostly played by her music therapist on piano, gong and tuning forks. One therapist (Martha) and one client (Karen) talked about sessions with recorded classical music. Martha played classical records and Karen was surrounded by classical music in her GIM (Guided Imagery and Music) sessions with Beth.

General Characteristics of Meaningful Moments

All meaningful moments were experienced on multiple levels. Meaningful moments occurred on internal, intrapersonal levels, and on external, interpersonal levels. The music that was shared caused inner movements within the client and within the music therapist. These inner movements occurred within four realms: the physical realm, e.g., changes in body sensations, changes in facial expressions; the cognitive realm, e.g., changes of thoughts and ideas; the emotional realm, e.g., changes in feelings and moods; and the spiritual realm, e.g., getting in touch with the soul and having spiritual feelings and meanings.

All meaningful moments were difficult to describe. All music therapists and clients interviewed found it very difficult to verbally express these experiences. In a sense, there were no words that could accurately convey the inner experience on all the different levels. Observations about this difficulty in expression include:

> It's hard to know what to say about it (Lucy); I am struggling
> with the words (Beth); I recognize it when I am there, but to
> describe it, it's hard (Adam); It's hard to talk about intuition, I
> don't know . . . (Martha); I can't think of a word to describe it
> . . . I don't really know what to call it . . . I can't really think
> of the right word . . . (Kathy); It's hard to explain . . . (Lyn);
> I don't know what to say, it's really hard for me to put it into
> words . . . (Karen)

All meaningful moments happened spontaneously. All of these
moments were unexpected and unpredictable. The music therapist did not
plan these moments, but prepared the environment and was open to trust
himself and to receive whatever happened. It was true for the client as
well, who did not anticipate these moments. None of the clients had
specific expectations, but each was open to trust and receive whatever
happened. The only moment that existed was the "here and now."

Statements concerning these points were as follows:

> I never know where something is going to move to . . . There
> has to be a willingness to accept whatever it is that comes up and
> that we follow it (Lucy); I didn't plan for Sue to blow this horn,
> it wasn't one of my goals for her, but somehow I left these horns
> on the shelf (Beth); I can't say that I can plan it or have a goal
> or a strategy for that. I can say that I make myself available
> (Adam); I didn't even know where I was going; it was very,
> very spontaneous . . . it just happened. I was committed to
> seeing what is going to happen and where is it going to take me
> . . . and I didn't know that it would be like that (Kathy)

Meaningful Moments in the Music Therapy Process

There were twelve moments that occurred on an intrapersonal level:

1. *Moments of awareness and insight*: These were moments in which
a sudden awareness was accompanied by a new meaning and occurred
intuitively or intellectually.

2. *Moments of acceptance*: These were moments where the clients accepted and embraced themselves or a part of themselves in a manner unlike any before.

3. *Moments of freedom*: Moments that included a feeling of expansion, relief and being more at ease, resulting from a release of tension and letting go.

4. *Moments of wholeness and integration*: These were instants in which the clients experienced a feeling of being at one with themselves, accompanied by a feeling of peacefulness.

5. *Moments of completion and accomplishment*: These were moments when the music therapists felt that their efforts and explorations bore fruit and the clients felt proud and had a sense of achievement in their music making.

6. *Moments of beauty and inspiration*: These were moments when the therapists were inspired by their clients' beauty, courage and authenticity. Also, the clients experienced their own inner beauty and a connection to the beauty that surrounded them.

7. *Moments of spirituality*: These were moments in which clients and therapists felt connected to God, connected to their own soul and had some kind of mystical and sacred experiences.

8. *Moments of intimacy with self*: These were moments when clients and therapists reached a new, deeper level of intimacy with themselves physically, emotionally and spiritually.

9. *Moments of ecstasy and joy*: These were moments in which therapists and clients experienced excitement, delight, joy, and exhilaration during their musical journeys.

10. *Moments of anger, fear, and pain*: These were moments when the clients got in touch with difficult feelings and emotions and expressed them either musically or verbally.

11. *Moments of surprise*: Moments in which clients and therapists were surprised by the quality and the intensity of their own experience or their clients' experiences.

12. *Moments of inner transformation*: These moments occurred when the clients experienced a powerful change that deeply affected their lives. The change was accompanied by tremendous joy and excitement.

There were three moments that occurred on an interpersonal level:

1. *Moments of physical closeness between the therapist and the client*: These moments were experienced by music therapists. During these

moments, therapists had some kind of physical contact with their client that brought a feeling of closeness and intimacy.

2. *Moments of musical intimacy between the therapist and the client*: These moments were experienced by music therapists. During these moments, the therapist experienced a powerful musical connection with his client that brought a feeling of intimacy between the two and resulted in new musical adventures.

3. *Moments of close contact between the client and a significant person in his life*: During these moments, the client achieved a new level of intimacy with a friend, a brother and a wife.

Environmental Factors that Allowed these Moments to Come to Birth

Music. All of the clients and music therapists who were interviewed underscored the crucial importance of music in producing meaningful moments for both therapists and clients. The music gave clients motivation to take risks and opened up areas that were closed before. Music allowed them to experience new ways to relate to the world and to make a significant connection. Music gave them delight and joy.

Being part of a music therapy group. Two of the clients and two of the therapists' clients participated in group music therapy. The group created a supportive atmosphere and motivated its members to take risks and to try new sounds and new ways of being. The music that was played by the group gave the clients a chance to be a part of a bigger sound, part of a bigger piece. The group also allowed anonymity. In one case, the fact that the spotlight was on another child made it easier for the client to take a risk.

Therapists' Intrapersonal Factors that Allowed these Moments to Come to Birth

Therapists' knowledge and experience. Even though all of the moments happened spontaneously, they did not "just" happen by mistake. They resulted from many elements integrated together within each music therapist: knowledge, experience over the years and self-trust.

Therapists' listening to inner impulses, instinct and intuition. All music therapists reported the use of intuition, instincts and impulses in their work. There were two kinds of listening: listening to the self in order to gain an intuitive knowledge and at the same time listening to the client (to be described later). When the therapists acted on this type of intuitive knowledge it became an integral part of the work.

Therapists' listening and exploration of clients' needs. The client's needs became the essence of all the work. Being fully there with the client and continually listening were vital to the therapy. Constantly exploring the client's needs on all levels helped stimulate their growth and self-fulfillment.

Therapists' Trust. The therapists had to trust their knowledge, instincts, intuitions and impulses. They also needed to trust their clients and to have faith in the process since the future is always unknown.

Therapists' perception of the therapist-client relationship. All music therapists perceived their work as a joint journey. Both client and therapist traveled together to unknown places. To accomplish this, the music therapists fully accepted the clients and supported them in their journey.

Therapists' set of beliefs that influenced their work. The therapists' self-perception influenced these moments. Beliefs about personal growth contributed significantly to meaningful moments. For example, both Lucy and Adam perceived themselves as spiritual human beings doing spiritual work. This resulted in spiritual moments that both of them experienced in their work with some of their clients.

Clients' Intrapersonal Factors That Allowed these Moments to Come to Birth

Clients' meaning of music. It was the meaning that the client attached to the music that made it such an important factor. These musical moments allowed the clients to get in touch with their creative selves and most clients felt much more alive when they were making music.

Clients' view of self. The clients' self perception had a lot to do with their meaningful moments. For example, Karen's view of herself changed while being a music therapy client:

> It's the first time that I don't feel like I am a failure and I feel like I can do it. . . . In this GIM experience, even though there is a verbal part, I never felt that I wasn't doing it right.

The fact that she felt better about herself allowed meaningful moments to transpire. Other clients viewed themselves as creative human beings who needed to explore their creativity.

Clients' readiness, inner motivation, and commitment to the work. This category was shared by the clients interviewed and by the music therapists' perception of their clients. Therapists believed that the client needed to be ready for the work. The client had to be motivated to overcome neurological, emotional, physical and mental blocks through the music therapy process. The client had to be willing to share the journey with the music therapist and to be committed to the process of growth, although it was sometimes painful and difficult.

Clients' courage in taking risks. All music therapists agreed that their clients demonstrated courage. They risked trusting themselves and trusting their therapists. They opened up and tried new creative ideas to expand themselves. They showed parts of themselves that they had not shown before.

Clients' perception of music therapy as a special place. Clients perceived the music therapy sessions as a place where they could express their most intimate feelings. It was a place where they could learn about themselves and grow. It gave them the freedom to explore their own innovative, intuitive, creative process.

Clients' perception of the music therapist and the relationship between them. Each client perceived his\her music therapist as knowledgeable and intuitive. The relationship was an intimate one. This perception had a direct connection with the amount of trust each had in his\her music therapist. Therefore, the client's perception of the music therapist became a pre-condition to trust.

Clients' trust. Trust was a very important factor in contributing to meaningful moments. It was the underlying factor that permitted the clients to feel safe, secure, and able to take risks. The clients had to trust three elements: the therapists, themselves, the process.

The Role of The Process

It was the process that made the moments possible and the moments that made the process successful. The process bred familiarity and fueled trust. The clients were motivated to be more involved in the process, allowing them to take more risks and to experience success and delight.

The Contribution of These Moments to the Client's Life

Improved self-esteem. All of the clients interviewed reported powerful changes in their self-esteem. They strengthened their ability to take risks and to make important decisions in their lives.

Improved emotional and physical health. Some of the clients explained that they felt better emotionally and even physically after these moments.

Improved interpersonal relationships. Improved self esteem and a stronger sense of self brought a change in the clients' relationships with significant people in their lives as they reached a new level of closeness.

No improvement outside therapy. One music therapist (Beth) reported that she did not see any changes in her client, Mary, outside the music therapy room. This client was a non-verbal child who could not express herself and communicate her needs in any other way. Mary had a moment of connection and joy, but according to Beth, their progress was very limited. Beth reported that even though she did not see any noticeable changes outside therapy, the meaningful moments that Mary had during her music therapy sessions were "profound" and "priceless."

The Contribution of These Moments to The Therapist's Work and Life

Improved therapeutic skills. These were moments of awakening for the music therapists in the study, showing them how to work with their clients and knowing what direction to choose. They gained more self-trust and developed their intuitive self.

Personal Growth. All interviewed music therapists believed that the work contributed to their own personal growth. As a result of their clients' moments as well as their own moments in the process, they expanded themselves as human beings.

SUMMARY: METHODOLOGICAL CONSIDERATIONS

Me: The Researcher

Exploring intrapersonal aspects. The utilization of a qualitative method in both data gathering and analysis provided me with a deeper look into the intrapersonal experiences of clients and music therapists in this study. The qualitative analysis gave me the opportunity to analyze and to see beyond the external and obvious into the internal and unobvious elements of the music therapy experience. I believe that those who analyze various elements of music therapy and its effects on people exclusively in a quantitative way may miss the intrinsic power of music therapy.

Reporting the findings. Qualitative analysis also permitted me to report categories that derived from three participants only. For example, only two of the therapists' clients and one client interviewed provided data for the category "Moments of Acceptance." These moments were not reported by the rest of the clients interviewed, nor did they come out as the therapists' own moments. Yet, there was a strong rationale to include this category. First, acceptance proved to be a significant aspect of these clients' inner experience as perceived by their music therapists. Second, it could also be that I, as the human instrument, did not probe enough to see if the other participants had experienced this moment.

Using my whole self as a researcher. As a researcher, I used my whole self. I was able to use my intellect, intuition, instincts and impulses, feelings, physical sensations and years of clinical experience as tools to gain knowledge and insights.

Making the familiar unfamiliar. One of the most challenging aspects of this research for me was to make the familiar unfamiliar. Before I gathered data I had some sense of what the findings would be. Coming from a humanistic transpersonal perspective, I thought that all the moments would be healing and transformative ones.

However, while listening to, transcribing, and reading the first interviews, I realized with the help of my support group that in some places I was leading my interviewees in the directions I wanted them to go, thus imposing my own ideas on them. For example, when one of the therapists interviewed described her experience with her client, I felt that she had a feeling of oneness while playing the music with her client. When I introduced the word "oneness" to her and asked her if this was the way she was feeling, she said, "This is not a word I would use." After becoming aware of how I was directing the participants, I was able to let go of my preconceptions and let my participants convey their own experiences.

Acknowledging my own bias. When I first went through the data, the categories were clear and apparent to me—they were in the directions I hoped them to be, such as feelings of spirituality and joy. Again, I realized that the shaping of some of the categories was based more upon my insider's knowledge rather than on the unbiased reading of the data.

As I went on analyzing the data I realized that some of my intuitions and hunches were being confirmed and others were not. Not all of the meaningful moments were beautiful, transformative, joyful or exciting. I learned that some of the meaningful moments in a music therapy session were moments of anger, pain and frustration. The direction I was interested in as a researcher led me to explore the beautiful and joyful aspects of the music therapy experience. I focused less on other aspects of the experience that might be meaningful as well, such as ordinary, frustrating and incongruent moments between client and therapist. These aspects should be further looked at in order to get a more complete picture of the experience.

Personal development. This method helped me identify the most important aspects of music therapy and better understand the meaning of my own work as a music therapist. The constant re-shaping and refining of categories defined them in a clearer, more focused fashion. After finishing my research, I have been even more aware of the complexity of human beings and am awestruck by how far music can reach within a human being.

The Participants in the Study

Giving a holistic picture. The interviews enabled my participants to describe their experiences in a holistic manner. They used their own words and concepts in ways they felt were most suitable to express and clarify their meaning. For example, one of the participants sang and played music for me at the end of the interview, feeling the music expressed more accurately what he meant.

Personal Development. Some of the participants gained new insights into their experiences while being interviewed. All participants seemed to enjoy being interviewed and most of them commented that they did not usually have opportunities to talk so openly about their experience.

Developing an authentic language for music therapy. An important aspect of this study was to examine how therapists and clients describe their experience in the music therapy process. Because I was interested in understanding the experience of the participants, it was inevitable that there would need to be a step in the research where an essentially musical experience would be translated into verbal language. Therefore, we have a process in which language was being generated to describe meaningful moments—a language grounded in the perception of music and in the whole experience which included the individual's full response to the music and to the moment. The fact that there is so much congruity among the observed categories and the language describing the experience of meaningful moments suggests that there is indeed a phenomenon which was common to the participants and which could be identified as meaningful moments.

This is only the first step toward developing a descriptive language for music therapy of phenomena that have all too often been dismissed because the language seems to not be grounded in anything "real." As this study has demonstrated, the language has been grounded directly in the experience of the music and the interactions with clients and therapists.

REFERENCES

Amir, D. (1992). *Awakening and expanding the self: Meaningful moments in the music therapy process as experienced and described by music therapists and music therapy clients*. Doctoral Dissertation, New York University. UMI Order # 9237730.

Bogdan, R. & Biklen, S. (1982). *Qualitative research for education*. Boston: Allyn & Bacon.

Ely, M. with Anzul, M., Friedman, T., Garner, D., & Steinmetz, A. M. (1991). *Doing qualitative research: Circles within circles*. New York: The Falmer Press.

Glaser, B. & Strauss, A. (1967). *The Discovery of Grounded Theory*. Chicago: Aldine.

Lincoln, Y. & Guba, E. (1985). *Naturalistic inquiry*. Beverly Hills, CA: Sage.

Lofland, J. & Lofland, L. (1984). *Analyzing social settings* (2nd ed.). Belmont, CA: Wadsworth.

Spradley, J. (1979). *The ethnographic interview.* New York: Holt, Rinehart & Winston.

Strauss, A. L. (1987). *Qualitative analysis for social scientists.* New York: Cambridge University Press.

Fusion and Separation: Experiencing Opposites in Music, Music Therapy, and Music Therapy Research

Mechtild Langenberg
Jörg Frommer
Michael Langenbach

An experience of analytical music therapy of a single case is analyzed in this qualitative research project. The act of improvisation brings forth a musical product between patient and therapist which can be described as an experience of polarity. The patient's tendencies toward regression and fusion become more volatile, potent, and aggressive, thus showing a process of separation and individuation.

In this case study, typical relationship patterns of a narcissistic personality disorder are illustrated. Interruptions of dialogue experienced in the movement of contrasting feelings in music are analyzed in our ongoing research project. The model is developed to illustrate the experiencing of polarities in music improvisation and in relationships.

Music therapy practiced in the context of psychotherapy derives from the artistic medium of music itself and from its use in relationship-oriented improvisation. In this specific situation, movement is brought about by the tension caused by alternating between processes of bonding and processes of separation native to the medium of music.

The therapuetic process provokes mutual identification when dealing with tension in the area of regression or progression. This requires the application of an elaborated psychotherapy process such as analytically oriented music therapy, in which the specific act (encounter in an improvisation) is expanded to form the model of treatment. We have illustrated the principles of unity and separation as an "experience block" in a previous publication, displaying qualities of fusion and separation (Langenberg, 1988).

Sound and relations in music take shape within time; the encounter is heard and felt by the participants involved. "The sequence of tones energizes this form, making this musical shape radically different from other, more static forms" (Klaes, 1934, p. 34). Because the elements in music are constantly changing, one can illustrate the subjective experience of this process in the experience of time. Klaes coined the expression "present time," meaning the specific way music is experienced as a way to understand successive forms, a way of connecting the concepts "just now - now - later." These ideas, in their application to music, are grounded in Gestalt and holistic psychology (Wertheimer, 1963; Köhler, 1933). With this background one can therefore say that tones induce polarity and order time.

In his recent approach to music therapy research, David Aldridge (1992) compared the holistic character of musical perception with the earliest forms of communication which are subjected to powerful physiological and psychological influences. The relationship between musical and biological forms seems to suggest the holistic nature of humans and how they are composed in the world (Aldridge, 1992).

Analytical Music Therapy, a psychotherapy form applied to different clinical populations, is based on active music therapy, the concept of Mary Priestley. Beginning with a musical improvisation, the encounter and relationship between patient and therapist (with an individual or in a group setting) takes form. The patient can explore his or her own unconscious issues and memories, experience old and new types of relationships, experience and recognize feelings and emotions, and integrate realizations of primary and secondary processes in the interplay of music and speech (Priestley, 1975; 1980; 1983). Eschen (1982, 1983) broadened this method, recognizing the importance of associative improvisation and supervision in the training of music therapists and the establishment of an accredited academic course of study in music therapy.

As the practice of analytically informed music therapy (Langenberg, 1988) became more professional in Germany, music therapy was able to take on the function of an independent psychotherapeutic treatment within the framework of an integrated overall treatment plan (Heigl-Evers, Henneberg-Mönch, Odag, & Standke, 1986). In our experience, patients with serious relationship disorders and whose problems lie in the area of symbiosis and individuation can benefit most from this form of music psychotherapy. Musical improvisation is a perfect expressive form to draw attention to their tendency to sever contact in the middle of dialogue (Heigl-Evers, Heigl, & Ott, 1993).

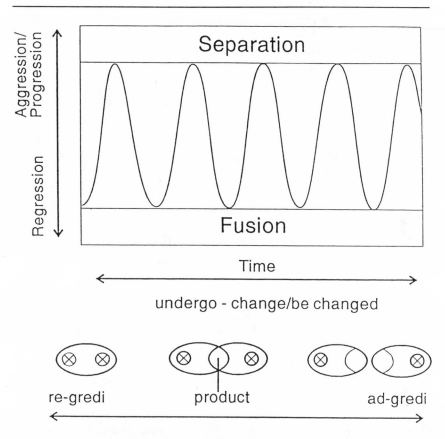

The image of an intersection illustrates the process clearly: it is dynamic, very alive, and can range from extremes of symbiosis to total separation. The image is ideal because the separate parts include the individuality of the various players and the whole, in addition to the individual quality of the particular encounter. The term "re-gredi" is Latin for regression and "ad-gredi" translates as aggression. The latter is used here in two senses: one that implies a confrontation that is conflict-laden and a second that merely implies the facing of another with one's separateness or autonomy. Langenberg (1988) elaborates further on these concepts.

Figure 1. Illustration of the process of experiencing fusion and separation during musical improvisation in a music therapy treatment situation.

The patient relives earliest experiences of relationships in the oscillation between primary and secondary processes which resembles a daydream-like condition; he can experience and order his splintered emotional world and distance himself from symbiotic and regressive experiences in the past.

Before beginning an improvisation, the patient is told the following: *Let us play whatever comes to mind, letting ourselves be guided by whatever needs to be expressed.* The basic rule of each session leaves room for the patient to experience qualities of the processes of bonding and separation, supported by the active involvement of the therapist who provides resonance by accompanying the improvisation.

The joint musical improvisation is an essential part of this approach. The vivid process of encounter and relationship in the music resulting from this method can be reheard and thereby relived and understood. Listening to a recording of the improvisation can help the listener perceive feelings, fantasies, images, etc. For the therapist, these are all indications that the listener is reliving internalized interpersonal experiences and conflicts from earlier developmental phases. The unconscious subject of dynamic psychotherapy becomes observable in the transference relationship of the therapeutic setting. An additional aspect in music therapy is that through direct resonance and common improvisation the material of the transference relationship is audible.

In order to grasp this differentiated interaction, methods appropriate to the material are required which do justice to the holistic character of this therapy process, a process with its own structures and meanings. This is also true in the field of psychotherapy research where researchers are currently calling for a more differentiated approach to case study research. In addition, they suggest that several models of describing psychotherapeutic processes should be tried out on a limited number of cases in order to be able to make statements about the effectiveness of these methods (Tress, 1988; Grawe, 1988; Tress & Fischer, 1991; Frommer, Hempfling, & Tress, 1992; Tress & Frommer, 1995). In this context, we developed the qualitative method of describing and interpreting works produced in music therapy treatment (Langenberg, Frommer, & Tress, 1992).

In analytically oriented music therapy, the individuals involved make use of a personal instrument known as the "resonator function" to relate to the other person (Langenberg, 1988). This concept includes the connotation of a musical instrument, as well as the capability to resonate and to be audible and tangible in the encounter. Additional qualities of the transference relationship become more apparent in music therapy.

In the music therapy encounter, the therapist is continuously available so that patient can directly experience periods of fusion and separation in the safety of musical play. We take advantage of this perceptive approach to explore the situation. In this way, we use a common approach for both the object and the procedure of recognition (Lorenzer, 1983). We regard the researched material involving the resonator function as a response to the work produced in treatment.

THE DÜSSELDORF PROJECT: QUALITATIVE RESEARCH OF IMPROVISATIONS IN MUSIC THERAPY TREATMENT

Attempting to integrate perspectives and approaches of qualitative social research into music therapy and music psychology (Gembris, 1991), we take advantage of the fact that the descriptions we received consist of relatively unstructured verbal material, similar to narrative interviews (Schütze, 1983). This allows for an interpretive and comparative evaluation. In general, when interpreting the texts we assume first that the background for the interpretation consists of subjective viewpoints and experiences of the individuals researched (Bergold & Breuer, 1987); second, that the categories in which the material is organized should be induced from the research material itself, becoming more abstract step by step (Strauss, 1987); and third, that the results of the interpretation stem from the comparison of data from various perspectives (triangulation) (Denzin, 1970; Flick, 1991). We use methods borrowed from the field of comparative case studies (Jüttemann, 1990) for the comparison of data.

Figure 2 shows our research design for the analysis of a music therapy session. Therapist and patient wrote down descriptions of the improvisation according to the instructions listed above. Afterwards, the recording was sent to four independent observers who wrote their own descriptions of the improvisation. In addition, a musical analysis of the improvisation was carried out, using an individual system of signs, similar to those used in the notation of contemporary music (Karkoschka, 1966). Last, these results were analyzed in relation to the clinical data from the patient's case history.

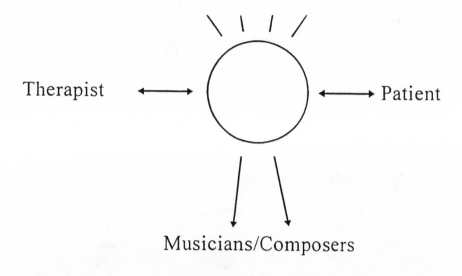

Figure 2. Triangle perspective related to the different levels of description. Independent describers, patient, and therapist receive the following instructions: *"Describe in a frank manner the associations that arise in you upon hearing the music. You can report feelings, thoughts, images, mental pictures, and stories, even if they seem chaotic."*

We developed the two general categorical dimensions of qualities and motifs, using ideas from a previous prototypical case (Langenberg, 1988; Langenberg, Frommer, and Tress, 1992).

Qualities

The term *qualities* is used to differentiate between content and subjective comments in the descriptions. All passages in the accounts that can be perceived as a response to the question: Which structures did I perceive in the content of the improvisation? are designated as *Quality 1*. Because the improvisations do not consist of verbal material, their descriptions are not direct, but comprise metaphors and mental imagery.   The improvisation, as a rule, is a gestalt, a process involving development of a holistic nature. Therefore, descriptions in the form of stories illustrating the procedural character of the music, are also appropriate. Quality 1 sums up all content, images, and scenes in a particular description.

Passages in the accounts that respond to the question: What did I feel? are designated *Quality 2*. With this designation we attempt to illustrate our experience that the descriptions convey how the listeners experienced the music, including the feelings evoked by or expressed in the music. These are closely related to statements expressing how the experience is related to the value system of the listener. Additionally, abstract, reflective thoughts about the material also belong to Quality 2. Thus, Quality 2 consists of the feelings, values, and reflections brought to mind by listening to the improvisation.

In a special list, which we call *Quality 2a*, we notated passages responding to the question: What feelings did this recording produce in me? This quality includes all the emotions, moods, values, and reflections that the describers do not use to describe the music, but designate as personal reactions to experiencing the music. Only in the patient's description of the improvisation did we choose not to differentiate between Quality 2 and Quality 2a.

Motifs

The next step in the evaluation process consists of a conclusive editing of the text material in an attempt to discern thematic categories which we call *motifs*. The process of qualitative content analysis (Mayring, 1983) aids us in methodically summarizing a *corpus*, rendering it more comprehensible. There are a variety of reductive strategies used in this analysis: omittance (statements that appear more than once are omitted); generalization (statements that are implied by more abstract statements are omitted); selection (central statements are retained unchanged); and, bundling (statements with closely related content, but found in various places in the text, are brought together as a whole).

In contrast to the approach used by Mayring (1983), we did not structure the reduced material according to previously fixed criteria, but rather in a way we called *open coding* (Strauss, 1987). We noted the thematic areas found in the text in a summarized form, working step by step through the material. An evaluation of this type was carried out for each of the descriptive texts.

The next step used methods borrowed from inter-individual comparative case studies (Jüttemann, 1990). Similar statements from the various descriptions (those of patient, therapist, and four to five independent describers) were placed in proper relation to each other in a table. We searched the material very carefully, looking for similar statements among the texts. Each motif then received a quote-like title. By evaluating the ratings in group discussions (Dreher and Dreher, 1991), we have attempted to reduce to a minimum the unavoidable influence of the subjectivity of the person performing the analysis native to such hermeneutic procedures.

The results of our first case study using this qualitative method have been published in previous articles (Langenberg, Frommer, and Tress, 1992; 1995). In this case, we illustrated the connections between motifs found in the text and aspects in the patient's biography, psychodynamics, and treatment.

We believe that our method is not only applicable to individual case studies, but also for the comparative study of patients with differing diagnoses. In the following section, we will present another single case, but in comparison to the above-mentioned patient, who suffered from chronic migraine headaches, we present here a patient with narcissistic personality disorder, displaying typical abrupt interruptions in dialogue and typical idealization and devaluation. Additionally, we will introduce another facet of our method in the context of this prototypical case.

After structuring the descriptive material by analyzing its contents according to our categories *Quality 1, 2, 2a*, and *Motifs*, we were further interested in the formation process each description underwent regarding the question: What process does the describer experience when he or she acts, as requested, as a resonator? What do the two individuals experience who are involved in the production of the music? What do the gradual formation process and their sequential structures, look like?

In order to answer these questions, we decided to examine the order in which the various motifs appear in the descriptions. It is our hypothesis that a form, a gestalt, becomes definable in the course of experiencing the music, in which the basic problem of the patient is mirrored, this being a fixation on mutually exclusive opposites. Closely related is the question: Can these expected rigid antimonies be somewhat loosened in order to make possible a dialectic process during the therapy session?

THE MUSIC THERAPY TREATMENT OF
MR. E: A CASE STUDY

We analyzed an improvisation taken from the course of music therapy treatment of Mr. E. using the research design explained above. Four independent persons, uninformed about the case at hand, reacted to the taped improvisation through the resonator function and recorded their personal reactions to what they heard. The patient and therapist also wrote down their associations using the same approach directly after the therapy session. A composer prepared a musical analysis of the recording.

Figure 3, on the following page, shows the description by the first person requested, including a summary of key words and our arrangement according to the various qualities.

Figure 4, on pages 141-143, shows the other descriptions; for reasons of space, we have not included the arrangement of key words according to qualities.

A general overview of the motifs, according to their respective texts, can be found in Table 1, pages 144-145. All of the texts contain references to a condition that suggests, if remotely, the gentleness of a mother to her child. Feelings of comfort and harmony are just as important as are aspects of being cared for or of symbiotic clinging to the mother (*I Nest motif*). Ambiguous, noncommittal aspects were also found in all of the texts (*II Pretense motif*), as well statements of intended separation, achieved via great tension in the music (*III Separation motif*).

Three of the descriptions, not including those of the patient and therapist, spoke of the experience as a performance (*IV Stage motif*). Further, motifs of power and strength appear in imagery of destruction or strife (*V Strength motif*). We found a climax similar to a dramatic development in three texts, including that of the therapist, not however that of the patient (*VI Development motif*). All describers perceived characteristics of weakness in their fantasy figures and stories and made mention of wanting to retreat or give up. Also reported was the feeling that something is missing (*VII Weakness motif*).

Text 1

For the most part, I found the music pleasant and relaxing,
something between a sound game and meditation. I had a fantasy
of a very close, harmonious, or harmoniously intended (unsure
which) togetherness. The person who is not playing piano
reacted to each impulse immediately. It is very dense. Sometimes
I have difficulty telling the players apart, or perceiving each
separately. The pianist's short-lived attempts to abandon the
harmony are ignored. Evidently discordant notes are not
allowed. Sometimes there is an uncertain, barely audible
scratching in the background, that doesn't match the rest of the
music at all. I am not sure if it is being played or if it is a
problem with the recording.

Quality 1	Quality 2	Quality 2a
person not at piano reacted to each impulse immediately	intended harmony (unsure)	music pleasant, relaxing - between sound game and meditation
background uncertain	very dense, short-lived attempts by the pianist to give up the harmony are ignored - discordant tones not allowed	close, harmonious
scratching		togetherness
	barely audible	difficult telling the players apart - perceiving each separately
	doesn't match rest of music	
	recording	not sure if it is being played

Figure 3. Description by the first independent listener; organization of
the text according to key words and structure according to qualities.

Text 2

<u>Circus ring</u>

* clowns playing their tricks
* acrobats in action
* jugglers throwing balls and pins into the air
* soap bubbles rise and pop
* then suddenly, the "strongest man on earth" appears
* the cheerful, colorful scene becomes a threatening scenario
* the artists, then the audience, panic
* all flee, except for the strong man who remains in the ring, showing off his muscles with an evil look on his face
* little by little, his activities become less threatening and more helpless, expectant
* all others return to "get him back on his feet again," but this doesn't work
* a sad, oppressive atmosphere remains

Text 3

Extremely mixed, broken impressions. In general, the piece is far too long; it could have been ended with the rather tender phase during which I had images of snow falling silently, calm and peaceful. That must have been about the middle of the piece. At first, images of a winter landscape, then a desert, then winter landscape again. Very melodic, the piano in the foreground, pleasant, harmonious, warm. The patient hardly stands out, which doesn't bother me at all. I abandon myself to these peaceful harmonies. Then, increasing, becoming louder, with the beats of the cymbal reminding me of a mountain slope in winter, an avalanche in the background, restless feeling in my stomach. Yet the music is not uncomfortably loud; it just goes all through me, rather thrilling. However, no manifested fear in me, but a

Figure 4. Descriptions of the second, third, and fourth independent listeners, and of patient and therapist.

very diffuse feeling of suspense. Then, again, sounds reminding me of Keith Jarret's concert in Cologne; I can ignore the scraping and rattling in the background; the piano clearly dominates—pleasant to hear. Then the tender music mentioned above, a very caring touch, just like a mother holding her child tenderly in her arms, stroking and caressing it. Thoughts of a loving closeness, almost symbiosis. But the child, the patient, won't stop. It starts to become irritated; the piece refuses to come to an end. Maybe I would have liked to listen to the piano further, but the background noise starts to bother me; at least that's how I see it. No more images, more thoughts, again a winter landscape, now leafless trees, several dead boughs. But no sadness, rather a feeling of suspense, and, as mentioned, irritation. Regarding the patient, all I could say is that the person may be shy; but when he strikes, the music becomes irritating. On the other side, his volume in the first third of the piece had a certain attraction. Like I said, it went all through me.

Text 4

Dewdrops, heavy rain, a person stamps through puddles, goes with his head bowed in the rain, opens a gate and goes across the wet pasture, does his work there, returns, closes the gate, goes home. He enters the house, where it is warm and dry. Silence falls. The man talks to his wife, and suddenly they are involved in a fierce argument, as if the storm were breaking inside the house; too much tension, suddenly discharged. An intense change of words, calming down, both parties try to keep their composure, to restore order, but old issues keep coming up, and the two hurt each other with injurious statements. A calm returns little by little; the heaving and raging sea comes to rest. Approaching the end, the music gets boring, and my thoughts stray to my own problems.

(Figure 4, continued)

Patient

Today's improvisation was an expression of my sensuousness. With all its peaks and valleys it expressed the spectrum of my sensory impressions. The whole time, I had the feeling that I was with myself. In me, with me, and not alone. Only the end was missing . . . When does sensuousness end and aggression begin?

Therapist

Again, there is immediately a very close understanding and spectrum of variation between us. From a very joyful, rising music to quiet, childlike melody forms that make me smile. It is simply a joy to play with him; he seems to enjoy it as well, and occasionally we exchange glances. Then, the music seems to become more serious; the patient tries, increasingly, to become more prominent and explosive. The mutual stimulation appears to approach a climax. Again and again, the music becomes shrill, which is fun, but it never gets to discharge. Finally, the patient pulls his music back and stops the tones—I also pull out and expect the end of the music. A new encouraging impulse comes, accompanied by strengthening glances, and again I play, too. Increasingly I wonder how this will come to a resolution, since new impulses to keep playing come constantly from the patient, and since this is our last session. More and more I hold myself back and listen to his movements; finally the cymbal resounds with one strike, while I repeatedly play the note "A".

(Figure 4, continued)

Table 1. Overview of identified motifs in their distribution in the individual accounts.

Motifs	Patient	Therapist
I Nest	sensuousness (2) in me; with me—and not alone (2)	very close understanding (2); quiet childlike melody (2); constant new impulses to keep playing (2)
II Pretense	when does sensuousness end and aggression begin? (2)	never gets to discharge (2)
III Separation	aggression (2); peaks and valleys (2); end is missing (1)	more prominent and explosive (2); shrill (2)
IV Stage		
V Strength		
VI Development		from joyful to childlike (2); more serious music (2); approaching climax (2)
VII Weakness	ends when . . . begins when? end is missing (2)	quiet and childlike (2); no discharge (2); hold myself back (2a)

Table 1, continued

Text 1	Text 2	Text 3	Text 4
reaction to each impulse increasing harmony (1); difficulty telling players apart (2a)	cheerful, colorful, scene (2); back on his feet again (2)	calm and peaceful (2); mother holding child tenderly in her arms (2); won't stop (2)	warm, dry, silence falls (2)
between soundgames and meditation (2a); intended harmony (2); not allowed (2)	soap bubbles rise and pop (1)	extremely mixed, broken impression (2); doesn't bother me at all (2a)	trying to keep composure and restore order (2)
ignore giving up of harmony (2); discord (2); scratching does not match	threatening scenario, panic (2); all flee (1)	piece refuses to end (2); avalanche (1); background noise (2a); irritating (2)	argument (2); storm (2); injurious statements (2); too much tension (2)
background (1)	circus ring (1)	concert in Cologne (1)	
	strong man (2), show off muscles (1)	piano clearly dominates (2); when he strikes (2)	fierce argument (2); storm (2); heavy, raging sea (2)
	cheerful, colorful scene becomes threatening scenario (2)	winter landscape, desert, again winter landscape (1)	calm, argument, storm (2); work, house (1)
ignore (2); discordant tones are not allowed (2)	helpless, expectant (2); doesn't work (2); sad, oppressive atmosphere (2)	shy (2); dead boughs (1)	old issues come up (2); bowed head (2)

Table 2. Overview of all motifs found in the chronological order they appear in the descriptions.

Text 1	Text 2	Text 3
Nest (2a)	Stage (1)	Pretense (2)
Pretense (2a)	Strength (1)	Separation (2)
Nest (2a)	Pretense (1)	Nest (2)
Pretense (2)	Strength (2)	Nest (2)
Nest (1)	Nest/	Development (1)
Nest (2)	Development (2)	Development (1)
Nest (2a)	Separation (2)	Nest (2)
Separation	Separation/	Weakness (2)
/Weakness (2)	Weakness (1)	Pretense (2a)
Separation/	Strength (1)	Nest (2a)
Weakness/	Stage (1)	Strength (2,1)
Pretense (2)	Strength (1)	Pretense/
Stage (1)	Strength (2)	Stage (1)
Separation (1,2)	Weakness (2)	Separation (1)
Weakness (2a)	Nest (2)	Strength (2a)
Pretense (2, 2a)	Weakness (2)	Strength (2a)
	Weakness (2)	Stage (1)
		Separation/
		Pretense (2a)
		Strength (2)
		Nest (2), Nest (2)
		Nest (2), Nest (2)
		Separation (2)
		Separation (2)
		Separation (2)
		Pretense (2a)
		Development (1)
		Weakness (1)
		Strength (2)
		Separation (2)
		Weakness (2)
		Strength (2)
		Separation (2)
		Strength (2a)

(Table 2, continued)

Text 4	Patient	Therapist
Strength (1)	Nest (2a)	Nest (2)
Weakness (2)	Strength (2a)	Strength (1)
Development (1)	Nest (2a)	Development (2)
Strength (1)	Weakness/	Weakness/
Development (1)	Separation (2a)	Nest (2)
Nest (2)	Separation/	Nest (2a)
Development (2)	Strength 2a)	Pretense (2)
S e p a r a t i o n /		Nest (1)
Strength (2)		Development (2)
Separation/		Separation/
Strength (2)		Strength 2
Nest (2)		Development (2)
Pretense (2)		Separation (2)
Weakness (2)		Nest (2)
Separation (2)		Weakness/
Nest (1)		Pretense (2)
Strength (2)		Development/
Nest (2)		Separation (1)
Weakness (2a)		Weakness (2a)
		Strength (2)
		Nest (2)
		Separation (2a)
		Nest (2)
		Separation (2a)

In our previous research, the categorical dimension of the motifs help reveal important thematic areas in the production and experience of musical improvisation. Until now, however, we had not examined to what degree the dynamics of the experience, which are constantly changing, influence the encounter and relationship process. We illustrated a part of these dynamics by determining their classification according to qualities.

The distance in Quality 1 allows the describer to project the experience in stories or forms onto something other than himself. Quality 2 comes closer to the describer's own intrapsychic experience and Quality 2a includes the describer's most personal resonance.

The change and motion in these processes become more distinct via the newly introduced facet of our method. While Table 1 shows a general index of the motifs, Table 2 is an illustration of the motifs in the chronological order in which they appear in the descriptions. The changing states of experience of the describers and producers of the improvisation (patient and therapist), when seen in their sequential structure, describe a course of development. Each person who comes in contact with the music perceives a typical successive form that expresses his or her own subjective perspective of the experience, the perception of the passage of time being an important characteristic of music. Going through this process means changing and being changed; the motifs appear to be in motion between regressive and aggressive or progressive states of being. The dialectic processes derived from the descriptive material have been grasped in motion. In each description, we were able to illustrate what the describer underwent while listening to the recorded music, what states of being, what contradictory conditions (Fischer, 1989) he experienced in the course of listening. These processes can be compared to the course of development in the written descriptions of the persons involved in producing the improvisation.

The text material illustrates the describers' experiences as they recall them, in the sequence they appear. The subjective access to the experience, just as in the retelling of a dream, determines the form of a primary process. Our interpretation below is an attempt to grasp, hypothetically, the meanings of various sequences.

The *first describer* begins with the Nest motif (which receives a personal meaning in Quality 2a), questions this condition twice via the Pretense motif, and then attempts to separate from the motif. This becomes visible in passages in the text, double or triple coded as Separation/Weakness and Separation/Weakness/Pretense, leading to the possible conclusion that the listener experiences separation as a condition of weakness in these passages. Via the Stage motif, which also appears in the "reserved" Quality 1, and a renewed attempt at separation, the first describer's resonance comes to an end in a condition of personal weakness and pretense (Quality 2a).

The *second describer* begins with the Stage motif and remains in the Strength and Pretense motifs in the "reserved" Quality 1. As he experiences the state of power, he seems to get more personally involved with the experience (Quality 2) and perceives a change to the Nest motif, related to development. Via the Separation motif, his state of being returns from the emotional Quality 2 to Quality 1 in the motifs of Separation, Power, Weakness, through the Stage motif to Power again, where he again returns to Quality 2 and remains there until the end, with the accompanying emotional states of Weakness, Nest, and twice at the very end, Weakness.

In the long text of the *third describer*, the experiential states begin in the emotional Quality 2, starting with Pretense and continuing on via Separation to Nest, where the describer remains before experiencing a more reserved development to Quality 1. He then returns to the Nest motif, experiences Weakness, Pretense, and again the Nest character, this time even in the intimate Quality 2a. The description continues with the Strength motif, a double code Pretense/Stage, and then goes on via Separation to a very intense experience of the Strength motif, recounted twice in Quality 2a. Then, the Stage motif follows, a double code Separation/Pretense, and Strength, returning then to a long phase involving the Nest motif (four times in Quality 2). The resulting condition of experience alternates between Weakness and Strength motifs until the end, where the describer is touched in Quality 2a.

The text of the *fourth describer* begins with the Strength motif in Quality 1, then moves through Weakness (Quality 2), Development (Quality 1), Strength (Quality 1), Development (Quality 1) to the Nest motif, touching the describer personally (Quality 2). Then comes Development (Quality 2), followed by the double code Separation/Power (Quality 2), which is reinforced twice. The describer then tends strongly in a regressive direction, before ending intimately with the Weakness motif in Quality 2a.

It is conspicuous in Table 1 that neither the patient nor the therapist experiences the Stage motif. The patient also does not experience the

Development motif, which is, however, mentioned by the therapist and three describers. This could point to differences between the *on-line-perspective* of the therapist and the client on the one hand and the *off-line-perspective* (Moser, 1991) of the independent describers. The latter may be bringing in critically some unfinished business of the therapy; they may be perceiving possible aggressive aspects of the client-therapist interaction which are denied by the actors of the therapy. These, however, are held at an impersonal distance by the constantly recurring stage-like atmosphere.

The *patient*'s gestalt process (Table 2) begins with the Nest motif. At first, he experiences strength, then describes a motion or change in the double codes Weakness/Separation and Separation/Power, which could be interpreted as a successful attempt to move from a very intensive, regressive state, in which separation sets free feelings of weakness and strength, in a more progressive direction.

Last, the *therapist* experiences the beginning of the encounter similarly to the patient. She differentiates the motions in greater detail, expressed in the longer text and double codes that point to the ambivalence of the state of separation (Weakness/Nest, Separation/Power, Weakness/ Pretense, Development/Separation). A state of separation dominates the end, illustrating the alternating regressive and progressive movement, which is experienced very intensely (Quality 2a). The motifs of Nest (Quality 2) and Separation (Quality 2a) mark the close of the improvisation.

The therapeutic process in this treatment period is following a dramaturgy involving intense acts of fusion and separation. There are attempts at separation from the extreme unity represented by the nest character which is an image of intimacy and dependence; these attempts involve a wide spectrum of dynamic possibilities, as well as unclear pretenses and staged dramaticism. In all of the gestalt processes of this therapeutic interaction the interplay of contradictory states and conditions plays an important role. In the music, counteracting forces develop in fantasies; these may appear unconnected on the primary process level, but during the process of therapy these fantasies can become connected with each other.

A "Musico-graphic" Perspective

Listening to an audiotaped piece of music from a therapy session is similar to reading the transcript of a verbal psychotherapy session. It is, however, similar only in a certain way. One cannot *read* this kind of recorded material, one has to listen to it. Many listeners are able to get to grips with a piece of music by just listening. However, with time we tend to forget important individual particles and components of something we have just heard, unless we are gifted with a very good musical memory and a sound associative sense of accumulative comparison. This problem can be diminished only slightly by listening repeatedly to a musical work.

In research, most methods of assessing and evaluating a certain object rely on the free availability of that object so that one can review it repeatedly and at will for purposes of comparison and classification. In order to assess a music therapy session we can rely on listening and memorizing what we have heard. The evaluation process, however, can be helped by introducing a tool which is freely and continuously available, something which can be read and organized in a particular way.

To be able to "read" music, a set of transformations is required, a translation from something we can listen to into something we can read. Translation into another medium can involve the loss of something but has the advantage of looking at something in a different and new context.

By transforming music therapy sessions into verbal accounts by different listeners, the opportunity to place music within the context of other things we can talk about is provided. In particular, a verbal transformation offers the option to look at the full range of possible associations with music, such as connecting music with some vivid images, with emotional states or with particular events in people's lives. What a translation of music into words loses, however, has to do with some specificities of music. Music is a highly specific communicative medium which is difficult to define in its specificity. Wolfgang Rihm, a contemporary German composer defines music as "freedom, a sign-language of sound put on time, the trace of non-intellectual wealth of Gestalt . . . the sensuous expression of energy" (Eggebrecht, 1987).

The order of time and the sensuous, non-intellectual experience are perhaps the specific characters missed most in attempts at verbal transformation of music. We have tried, therefore, to add another perspective on the session under discussion which can be described as a musico-graphical perspective. The intention is to become more able to catch tensions, opposites, and specific features in their time order.

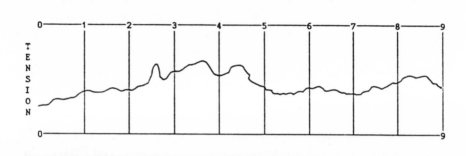

Figure 5. Musico-graphical perspective: Tension

The music is flowing smoothly. There is neither a structuring into smaller units, nor is there a sense of "movements" of a larger form. The character is that of a serenade or notturno, music to be played at night without dramatic eruptions. It is determined by its flow like a bubbling brook with two or three peaks. The whole work remains peculiarly aimless and vague at times. There are no abrupt changes initially, neither in instrumentation—except for the odd use of cymbal—nor in speed, character, or dynamics. The peaks develop over extended periods of time. One player is carrying the other one deeper into embracing a mutual musical figure which quickly becomes louder and more dense. The climax is characterized by the use of cymbal.

Then, the two partners withdraw again, suddenly, seemingly preoccupied with following their own musical thoughts until they start listening to each other again. They reach a second climax, even louder and more energetic than the first one, lasting a bit longer than the first one. Here, the two partners seem to confront each other with their musical material and to exchange ideas and feelings. Again, this climax does not endure for long, and the two players separate, forming musical fragments and brief sketches which do not relate to each other. The ending section is brief, without any conventional formula such as a cadenza or impressive cascades; it is rather casual. The piano tentatively stops playing and the metallophone carries on cautiously for a few seconds longer, and then stops too.

Looking at the music in more detail includes an overview of dynamics, density, color, tempo, cohesion, texture, and instrumentation in chronological order. Dynamics, density, and tempo of the music seemed to be important parameters for their direct relation to the energetic states of the players and to their emotional expression. Color was chosen as it appeared that some parts of the music were more warm and tender than others which sounded sharp and shrill. *Cohesion* is meant to describe the relation between the two players: how do they listen to each other, who is introducing a new theme, and so on, which seems to be an indication of the inter-relation of the two players. *Texture* looks at the lines and chords of the music: Is the music more linear, quasi-contrapuntal or more harmonic? The instruments used in this improvisation were piano, metallophone, and cymbal. The graphical signs make use of models used in modern music, e.g., signs used by A. Logothetis or John Cage (Karkoschka, 1961).

Comparing the musico-graphic perspective with the motifs of Table 1 we find indications to the character of the improvisation given by the resonator function of independent describers. The Nest motif can be found in the "carrying and embracing" atmosphere of the musical analysis and the seductive character. The Pretense motif is not there, but the Separation motif can be found in the description entailing: "withdraw, following their own musical thoughts, separate musical fragments." Aspects of the Strength motif are in "confront each other" and expressions like "energetic." The Development motif can be seen in the metaphor of the "bubbling brook," perhaps in the flowing character but obviously in "peaks develop." The motif of Weakness is analyzed by the musician as "aimless, cautiously, tentatively, vague at times."

The general character of the musical encounter perceived by a musician can be summarized in its primary aspects. There is a character of seduction to let go and give oneself away. The loving and tender aspects include an atmosphere of staying, aimlessness, and an absence of clear contrasting forms. Fusion and regression are strong impressions of delight. Why should there be separation when the two players enjoy being together so much?

Another central impression of the musical analysis is the flowing character as a typical element of making music which means the subjective experience of time and possibility of changing in experiencing polarities. The motifs as a response of the resonator function of listeners to the music gives a more static picture of the experience of this encounter. In the musico-graphic perspective we find now the possibility of movement and development. There are "no movements of a bigger form" but a search for contour and clarity in moving through different states and working on confrontation, exchange and separation.

The problem of differentiation and separation from each other is obvious but in progress. The end seems to be "casual," the encounter tentatively formed with sensuousness and little aggression in a sense of differentiation—power and strength. The separation is immature, young, in development, and touching.

A look at Table 2 with the sequences of motifs shows that the describers go through different states of experience similar to the patient and therapist who created the music. During the act of recreation, the

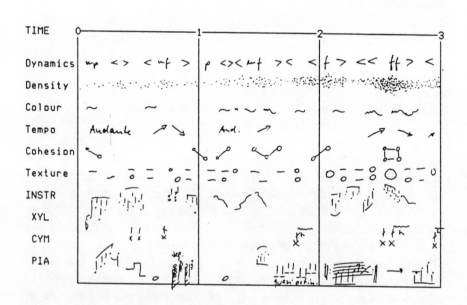

Figure 6. Musico-graphical perspective, dynamics, density, color, tempo, cohesion, texture, and instruments (Xylophone, cymbal, piano), first three minutes of the improvisation.

dynamics:	p piano	soft
	ppp pianissimo	extremely soft
	f forte	loud
	ff fortissimo	very loud
	fff forte fortissimo	extremely loud
	mp mezzo piano	medium soft
	mf mezzo forte	medium loud
	< crescendo	getting gradually louder
	> decrescendo	becoming softer

density:	the density of dots corresponds to density of sound

color:	round bows indicate soft, smooth flow
	sharp edges indicate forced accents

tempo:		increase of speed
		decrease of speed
	And(ante)	at a moderate speed
	Allegretto	lively
	Adagio	slow and broad
	poco sost(enuto)	sustained, in a smooth manner
	più mosso	more animated

cohesion:	motif of first player taken up by second player
	motif of second player taken up by first player

texture:	linear flow of music in chords

instruments:	xyl xylophone
	cym cymbal
	pia piano

abbreviations:	con sord.	with dampers
	(con sordino)	
	quasi ost.	persistently repeated musical
	(quasi ostinato)	figure

(Figure 6, continued)

listeners undergo a dramatic intrapsychic situation and experience states of polarity. Their effort to establish a clear, unambivalent perspective and contour can be seen in the double coding of some states of experience. In the musical graph, motifs overlap each other. For example, Separation can be experienced in combination with either Strength or with Weakness, indicating the subjective and personal experience of the particular resonator. In some cases, there are triple codings, such as Separation combined with feelings of Weakness and Pretense; in another sequence, there is development combined with Separation and Pretense. The new facet of describing and analyzing the improvisation via different resonators and perspectives depict the specific experiences of polarity.

In a previous study (Langenberg, 1988), the process of working out a conflict of ambivalence using dimensions of unity and separation was demonstrated. In this case study, it is our hypothesis that typical identification characteristics of a narcissistic personality disorder are pointed out in the evaluation of the various responses to the improvisation taken from the treatment. There is the all-embracing claim to be the center of everything, contradiction and paradox between strength and weakness are the focus of attention, and nuances and transitions seem to be missing at times. However, as the relationship comes into being, these develop from isolation to rough contact and to more fine-tuning and regulation of closeness.

To close, we will provide a few notes on the clinical aspects of our case study. The patient, a man, 33-years-old at the time of treatment, was suffering from disorders affecting his work and relationships. He described his symptoms as follows: feelings of insufficiency, social withdrawal, compulsive brooding, and somatic distress. Narcissistic and compulsive depressive aspects dominated his personality structure and there were significant problems with his self-esteem. The results of the last therapy session of an integrated overall treatment concept in a psychotherapeutic day hospital (Heigl-Evers et al., 1986) were evaluated and discussed. In this day hospital setting, the patient's individual therapy was in the form of analytically oriented music therapy.

The patient dramatized the discrepancy between his intellectual attitude and his great need for recognition by others to regulate his feelings of self-esteem. In this way, he was able to give up his verbal intellectual rivalry with others and to accept emotional closeness and vitality. The constant breaking-off of dialogue that initially appeared, accompanied by strong feelings and impulsive breakthroughs could be experienced and worked out in the fine-tuning framework of music therapy. The narcissistic way the patient dealt with himself and with the world led to constant feelings of being insulted and to broken-up relationships. Improving his self-perception and distinguishing among his feelings and expressions helped point out the discrepancy between reality and his fantasies of grandeur, thereby helping him to work out these problems.

SUMMARY

In researching works produced in music therapy treatment we are interested in understanding the feelings and thoughts involved in the interpersonal encounter that is the basis of improvisation. In this encounter, typical relationship patterns are repeated but the artistic medium of music improvisation, with its specific characteristics, offers the potential to experience and work through the conflicts embedded in these patterns. Our research has shown that opposites, on the one hand, can remain side by side like rival powers, to come to greater differentiation. On the other hand, movement, shaping, and change are experienced and integrated if the resonant space of our procedure is made use of.

The gestalt process, a new facet of our method, points to flexibility as an important factor in working out difficult problems with relationships and interpersonal contact. The patient is able to bond with and separate from others with less danger, because he has room to grow and develop in the space within the music with its primary and secondary process traits.

REFERENCES

Aldridge, D. (1992). Physiologische Veränderungen beim Spielen improvisierter Musik - Einige Vorschläge für Vorschungsarbeiten. *Musiktherapeutische Umschau, 3,* 174-186.

Bergold, J. & Breuer, F. (1987). Methodologische und methodische Probleme bei der Erforschung der Sicht des Subjekts. In J. Bergold & U. Flick (Eds.), *Einsichten. Zugänge zur Sicht des Subjekts mittels qualitativer Forschung.* Tübingen: DGVT-Verlag.

Denzin, N.K. (197O). *The research act.* New York: McGraw-Hill.

Dreher, M. & Dreher, E. (1991). Gruppendiskussionsverfahren. In U. Flick, E. v. Kardorff, H. Keupp, L. v. Rosenstiel, & S. Wolff (Eds.), *Handbuch Qualitative Sozialforschung.* München: Psychologie Verlags Union.

Eggebrecht, H.H. (1987). Gibt es "die" Musik? In C. Dahlhaus & H.H. Eggebrecht (Eds.), *Was ist Musik?* Wilhelmshaven: Noetzel, Heinrichshofen-Bücher.

Eschen, J. Th. (1982). Mentorenkurs Musiktherapie Herdecke, Ausbildung von Ausbildern. *Musiktherapeutische Umschau, 3,* 255 - 282.

Eschen, J. Th. (1983). Assoziative Improvisation. In H.H. Decker-Voigt (Ed.), *Handbuch der Musiktherapie.* Bremen: Bremen.

Fischer, G. (1989). *Dialektik der Veränderung in Psychoanalyse und Psychotherapie.* Heidelberg: Asanger.

Flick, U. (1991). Triangulation. In U. Flick, E. v. Kardorff, H. Keupp, L. v. Rosenstiel, & S. Wolff (Eds.), *Handbuch Qualitative Sozialforschung.* München: Psychologie Verlags Union.

Frommer, J., Hempfling, F. & Tress, W. (1992). Qualitative Ansätze als Chance für die Psychotherapieforschung: Ein Beitrag zur Kontroverse um H. Legewies "Argumente für eine Erneuerung der Psychologie. *Journal für Psychologie, 1,* 43-47.

Gembris, H. (1991). Musiktherapie und Musikpsychologie: Möglichkeiten einer interdisziplinären Kooperation. *Musiktherapeutische Umschau, 12,* 279-297.

Grawe, K. (1988). Zurück zur Psychotherapeutischen Einzelfallforschung. *Zeitschrift für Klinische Psychologie, 17,* 1-7.

Heigl-Evers, A., Henneberg-Mönch, U., Odag, C., & Standke, G. (Eds.). (1986). *Die Vierzigstundenwoche für Patienten: Konzept und Praxis teilstationärer Psychotherapie.* Göttingen: Vandenhoek & Ruprecht.

Heigl-Evers, A., Heigl, F., & Ott, J. (1993). *Lehrbuch der Psychotherapie.* Stuttgart Jena: Fischer.

Jüttemann, G. (Ed.) (1990). *Komparative Kasuistik.* Heidelberg: Asanger.

Karkoschka, E. (1966). *Das Schriftbild der Neuen Musik.* Celle: Moeck.

Klaes, A. (1934). *Studien zur Interpretation des musikalischen Erlebens.* Langensalza: Beyer und Mann.

Köhler, W. (1933). *Psychologische Probleme.* Berlin: Springer.

Langenberg, M. (1988). *Vom Handeln zum Behandeln: Darstellung besonderer Merkmale der musiktherapeutischen Behandlungssituation im Zusammenhang mit der freien Improvisation.* Stuttgart: Fischer.

Langenberg, M., Frommer, J. & Tress, W. (1992). Qualitative Methodik zur Beschreibung und Interpretation musiktherapeutischer Behandlungswerke. *Musiktherapeutische Umschau, 4,* 258-278.

Langenberg, M., Frommer, J. & Tress, W. (1995). From isolation to bonding. A music therapy case study of a patient with chronic migraines. *The Arts in Psychotherapy, 22,* 87-101.

Lorenzer, A. (1983). Sprache, Lebenspraxis und szenisches Verstehen in der psychoanalytischen Therapie. *Psyche, 2,* 97-115.

Mayring, Ph. (1983). *Qualitative Inhaltsanalyse.* Weinheim: Beltz.

Moser, U. (1991). Vom Umgang mit Labyrinthen: Praxis und Forschung in der Psychoanalyse - eine Bilanz. *Psyche, 45,* 315-334.

Priestley, M. (1975). *Music therapy in action.* London: Constable.

Priestley, M. (198O). Analytische Musiktherapie und musikalischer Respons. *Musiktherapeutische Umschau, 1,* 21-36.

Priestley, M. (1983). *Analytische Musiktherapie.* Stuttgart: Klett-Cotta.

Schütze, F. (1983). Biographische Forschung und narratives Interview. *Neue Praxis, 3,* 283-293.

Strauss, A.L. (1987). *Qualitative analysis for social scientists.* Cambridge: Cambridge University Press.

Tress, W. (1988). Ein Blick auf die Konturen des Elefanten. Bericht von der 19. Jahrestagung der Society of Psychotherapy Research (SPR) in Santa Fe vom 14. - 18. Juni 1988. *Zeitschrift für Psychosomatische Medizin und Psychoanalyse, 35,* 175-186.

Tress, W. &, Fischer, G. (1991). Psychoanalytische Erkenntnis am Einzelfall: Möglichkeiten und Grenzen. *Psyche, 45,* 612-628.

Tress, W. & Frommer, J. (1995). Beziehungspathologie und therapeutische Dyade. Ein Beitrag zur psychopathologischen Prädiktion von Ergebnissen dynamischer Psychotherapie. In M. Rösler (Ed.), *Psychopathologie: Konzepte - Klinik und Praxis - Beurteilungsfragen.* Weinheim: Beltz.

Wertheimer, M. (1963). *Drei Abhandlungen zur Gestalttheorie.* Darmstadt: Wissenschaftliche Buchgesellschaft.

PART II: DIALOGUES

The Researcher's Cultural Identity

Kenneth Aigen

> *We anxiously follow what we suppose to be important, while what we suppose to be unimportant wages guerilla warfare behind our backs, transforming the world without our knowledge and eventually mounting a surprise attack on us.*

> Milan Kundera
> *The Book of Laughter and Forgetting*

What is it important to know? How do we know what is important to know? These are the questions I would like to consider here, that I have been considering for the months preceding this writing. This dialogue consists of some tentative answers.

Consider this statement:

> As qualitative researchers we use our selves as the research instrument.

Although I have been aware of this throughout my tenure as a qualitative researcher, it has recently taken on more dimensions for me. This enhanced awareness of the implications of the researcher-as-instrument was stimulated primarily by interactions at the Symposium in Düsseldorf. I am offering these experiences and thoughts to contribute to the communal store of experience and to help consolidate and further my own development. This is the spirit in which this telling is undertaken.

Here is one aspect of my epistemology:

I believe what is told by the people I trust.

Of course, trust is established in many ways, often through personal contact. Yet in reading qualitative research reports we are often asked to trust those who we may never meet. In the absence of this contact I look for alternative ways of establishing trust, such as that the person demonstrates some capacity for self-knowledge and self criticism, and that the ideas presented are related to the larger web of life. I am writing this story in order to provide a context for my previous contribution to this volume and to tell some of the things I would say had I a personal contact with each person who might read this.

As is true for most people, I am part of many communities. One of these communities is just beginning to form and take shape. It is the community of music therapists interested in developing qualitative research approaches to better understand their clinical work, their clients, and themselves, and in communicating this enhanced understanding to others. A Symposium was organized by Mechtild Langenberg that represented a first gathering of the community, although there were historical precursors and the works of other related communities which enabled this gathering to occur. At this Symposium we were coming together not to share research results but to discuss how to do qualitative research and how to evaluate it. We defined ourselves as being more interested in the research process than in the research product for purposes of this gathering.

I was deeply affected by the personal interactions, by the process, at this meeting. I have been uncertain whether or not discussing the ways in which I was affected would be interesting to others and if these effects would be considered relevant to the purposes of this community and this book, and if friends and colleagues would be disturbed or offended by what I had to say. Yet my interactions with members of the community, particularly Carolyn Kenny, have convinced me of the importance of this discussion. I am the research instrument, as we all are, and to best understand the research one must understand the research instrument. This is also part of my epistemology, if you will, and the rationale for what follows.

Prior to arriving in Düsseldorf I was very eager to experience the feelings of colleagueship and community that I hoped would develop there. Yet, in the preceding months, I also had feelings of apprehension about coming to Germany. Being Jewish, I have always felt this reluctance on some level, although interactions with German music therapy colleagues and students have taken the edge from these feelings through time. What has happened for me is that the reality of coming to know German people has replaced the fantasy in my mind and helped me to begin to overcome my own hesitations. Nevertheless, I found it difficult to acknowledge that this trip was part of an internal process of overcoming fears and prejudices.

That the content of my talk at the Symposium was affected by these feelings points to the fact that, as researchers, we are also subject to the impact of human history. This is another sphere of influence that shapes who we are and that can distort our thinking or limit us if we are not cognizant of its forces. The past shapes and influences us all, as much as do the experiences through which we actually live.

Once arriving at the Symposium, however, these thoughts were not particularly active in my awareness. After the opening, I began the series of presentations used as a basis for discussion among the participants. I felt compelled to consider the issue of values; I was not sure why at the time although I was concerned that I not alienate colleagues who may have thought that I was trying to impose my values upon them.

The speaker following me was Henk Smeijsters. Part of his presentation concerned a comparison between quantitative and qualitative approaches. Henk is in a different place from me, believing that some of the standards of traditional research are essentially scientific and should be preserved when doing qualitative research. I was unclear as to why he was making the comparison when Henk made an honest admission: His thinking is in a process of development, it is time-bound, and it may change. This simple statement opened me to the points that Henk was making. This personal admission rendered me more able to *hear* him.

I was fascinated by the fact that such a simple, personal statement could help me to appreciate Henk's ideas in a different light. It strengthened my belief that the sharing of ideas is most productively done in a supportive context in which personal and professional considerations are integrated, and where the former are not only permitted but encouraged. I thought back one year to a previous conference where I had discussed a similar comparison in a presentation. I realized that at that time I had to say certain ideas publicly, both to consolidate them and to move on from them. Presenting these ideas put them into the communal debate and served to further my inner development.

All sharing of ideas has this dual aspect and when I listen to a colleague I can support the presentation because, while I may disagree with or not find the ideas compelling, I can support the inner growth that such public sharing facilitates. It is the forthcomingness of the presenter that activates my own capacity to be a supportive listener in this context.

Later in the Symposium, Kenneth Bruscia talked about his conception of the purpose of qualitative research which was to raise consciousness by bringing into our awareness what had previously been unconscious. I felt this happening at the Symposium as I was affected by the interpersonal process.

After Henk's presentation came that of Carolyn Kenny. Carolyn's discussion of the cultural influences upon her research and theory was most prominent for me. She attributed one of the sources of her clinical theory to her experiences in the Longhouse. About her work, she says that

> it is the story of who I am, where I have come from, my roots, where I belong. These memories help to form and shape my experience. If there are universal elements, they emerge from the dialogue with colleagues who I respect and can trust to reveal myself, in the sharing of human stories. (Kenny, 1996, p. 73)

What are my memories and roots? Where have I come from? How have these things shaped my ideas, particularly those that I just finished sharing with my colleagues? What is the story that I am living? Can I become aware of it? What of it will be of interest or of relevance to my colleagues? Carolyn's talk, her honesty, and her courage stimulated these questions in me.

Without formulating it in such terms, I was considering aspects of authenticity as the concept is presented by Kenneth Bruscia (1996) in Monologue 4:

> When I am authentic as a researcher, I bring into my awareness whatever is possible for me to bring into it regarding my study; I act in a way that is consistent with what is in my awareness; and I take appropriate responsibility not only for what is and is not in my awareness, but also for what I do not do in relation to it. (p. 82)

He further articulates that, for him, authenticity

> is an intrasubjective standard which governs the researcher's relationship to him/herself; it is not an intersubjective standard which governs relationships between the researcher, participant, phenomenon, and scholarly community. (p. 82)

This is an important consideration. It relieves us from the impossible task of becoming "authenticity police" judging fellow researchers. Yet, it places a greater responsibility on the individual to be the guardian of his/her own authenticity. I believe that Ken is correct in asserting that this is the foundational criterion for the other evaluative standards in qualitative research which are interpersonal in nature. As he succinctly observes, "How can I be trustworthy to other researchers, if I cannot trust myself as one?" (Bruscia, 1996, p. 82).

I felt challenged by these observations. I understood the notion of authenticity such that I am obligated to establish my authenticity to myself, not to others. Yet, I want to share my struggles in this area to help and encourage others on a similar path. I want to contribute to the community while simultaneously benefitting from the opportunity to have my struggles heard.

These efforts are important to me in order to act consistently with my beliefs. In Monologue 1, I say that

> our professional values should be *reflexive*, simultaneously applicable to the domain we are studying, our activities while conducting research, and the verbal and written forums in which we communicate with fellow researchers and present our findings. (Aigen, 1996, p.10)

Although Ken Bruscia does not argue for the extension of authenticity into other areas, if authenticity is one of the core values of qualitative research I feel compelled to manifest this value in all of my writings and interactions with the research community, not just in actually conducting research activity and reporting research results.

Into this maelstrom of ideas and emotions at the Symposium came Dorit Amir's presentation on her study of "Meaningful Moments in Music Therapy." Dorit spoke about how she came into her study with an interest in "meaningful moments" as an organizing construct, but felt compelled to hold this construct in abeyance when conducting and analyzing the interviews comprising the data of her study. Through her application of grounded theory data analysis, Dorit discussed how the concept of "meaningful moments" emerged from the data and became the fundamental construct organizing her data.

She was then questioned by Ken Bruscia as to why she did not ask people about their meaningful moments if this was her interest and the source of her study. Dorit explained that she wanted her theory to come from the participants, not just from herself. I responded to Dorit, saying that she had used selective sampling in choosing her participants. Because we acknowledge the influence of unconscious factors is it not possible that she pre-determined her findings by her selection of participants? I continued that Dorit could not have it both ways: the freedom to engage in purposive, selective sampling and the right to say that her constructs emerged purely from the data. My feeling was that it was more ingenuous to make a choice between the two and then own that choice.

At that point I stopped myself in the discussion of Dorit's work. Something was bothering me about my own agenda at the moment and I did not feel cleanly aware of my own motivations. I shifted my awareness to the level of group process and felt myself participating in an attack, albeit a mild one, on Dorit. I was addressing her and her work when instead I should be applying the same considerations to myself and my work. I was offering a critique and asking Dorit to own her choices without having done so myself! I began to feel that the group, with me as a central actor, was playing out some of its issues through Dorit.

I realized that although the debate arose in the context of Dorit's work, to be an authentic contributor I had to be careful not to unconsciously play out my inner debate in the guise of criticizing or analyzing Dorit's work. I then asked myself the question I asked Dorit: In the study, discussed in Monologue 1, I researched a group of developmentally-delayed adolescents in music therapy for one year. I presented as an important finding that the group followed the stages of rebellion, conflict and intimacy characteristic of groups of more fully functioning adults. Yet, I had deliberately selected this group for study because they were older and more verbal than others at the Clinic where I undertook the study, and because I knew that the two treating therapists had extensive experience in group process in music therapy. In other words, all of the reasons going into my selective sampling of this group could be seen as considerations which would make more likely the emergence of group process as a clinically significant factor.

At this point in the Symposium Carolyn Kenny and I engaged in dialogue and our talks helped me to perceive the group process and how I was participating in a scapegoating, of sorts, of Dorit. I could not help but be struck by the irony of this in light of my emerging feelings about the historical and personal context forming the background of the Symposium.

All kinds of conflicting feelings emerged for me then and subsequently. I had come to Germany with a vague, unnamed feeling of apprehension. I was being moved by my interactions with the participants and I was stimulated to self-reflection, both by Carolyn Kenny's honest discussion of her heritage and its effect upon her work and by Ken Bruscia's discussion of authenticity. The Symposium ended with me feeling in flux around all of these issues.

In the months between the end of the Symposium and the writing of this Dialogue, I continued to try to understand the impact of this experience. Carolyn Kenny talked extensively about one's ethnic identity as an appropriate context for understanding ideas and story. This has supported my next step which is the exploration of my own cultural identity and its relation to the ideas presented in Monologue 1 of this volume.

As Carolyn Kenny observes in discussing her Native American heritage, I feel that what follows are my memories of Judaism, how my identity has shaped my perception of the world and my decisions in it. I am not representing the objective reality of Judaism, just what I have taken from being part of its embrace.

I came to Germany to talk about values. But what are the sources of my own values and my interest in values? One of the primary ones is my cultural identification as a Jew. I am not particularly religious in the sense of participating in religious practices overtly. Yet the core values that guide my life are intimately connected to my Jewishness. Many of these came into play in my discussion of the role of values in music therapy research.

On a basic level, my love of music is connected to my Jewishness. It is this connection to the arts and a realization of their sacred function which has guided my life into music. Music speaks what cannot be spoken. As with any historically oppressed group, Jews have experienced much which cannot be spoken, one reason for our connection to music.

The discussion which closes Monologue 1 on the values that spring from music therapists' identity as part of the worldwide community of musicians is a transposition of my cultural Jewish identity into a more universal, multi-national, multi-tribe, multi-ethnic sphere.

The emphasis placed on social justice in Judaism has guided my life in many dimensions. In Monologue 1, this was manifested by an emphasis on pluralistic models of research in which participants and investigators are equals and participants are given a voice, not merely from methodological considerations but from ethical ones. Again, the Jewish experience has rendered us sensitive to the need to ensure that all voices are heard, not just those of the majority.

There is a strong role for the concept of *tzedakah* in Judaism, often translated as "charity" although this translation misses the emphasis on obligation that is part of the Jewish concept as I was taught it. Offering help to others is an obligation we incur as a condition of our existence as human beings. This emphasis on improving the world and the state of human beings in it was part of my decision to become a music therapist, a decision without which none of my thoughts in these areas would ever have been conceived by me.

Carolyn Kenny says that "systems reflect values, which reflect beliefs" (1996, p. 75). Or in reverse, our beliefs imply values which in turn create systems. I have chosen to write about values because of my belief that systems of research approaches are best understood in light of the values from which they are derived. Carolyn Kenny teaches that even more basic than these values are core beliefs. To follow the course of my own logic is to be committed to the exploration of fundamental beliefs which determine the values which in turn determine the research systems that we wish to follow.

To tie much of this together, to come full circle, consider Carolyn Kenny's statements that "native peoples believe in an intimate connection between the people and the land" and "our worldview is intimately connected to the land" (1996, p. 75). I relate intimately to these statements. While I have never felt connected to the land of my birth, New York, this connection is alive for me in three places: the desert areas of the Middle East, including the Negev desert in Israel and the Sinai peninsula; the four corners area of the American southwest (particularly northeastern Arizona); and the Olympic Peninsula of Washington state in the U.S. As a result, I understand the feelings Native Americans have toward the land. I have always felt an affinity between my Jewishness and my kindred feelings with some Native American cultures and part of this stems from common feelings on the relationship between a people and their land.

In addition to the connection between a people and its land, I believe that there is an intimate relationship between music and the land. Part of being born Jewish involves inheriting a longing and love for the land of Israel that has survived and been passed through many generations across thousands of years. It was this felt connection to the land which allowed Judaism to survive in spite of its diaspora. It is the feeling for the land and its relationship to music that figured in my reluctance to come to Germany.

In another work I have talked about a conception of music which came to me as a vision while under the stars in the high desert of Arizona:

> I began feeling the aliveness of my entire surroundings and imagined the various forms of life as actual sentient beings: I saw the trees as wise, old beings that had discovered a way to live in harmony with such a harsh environment. If only the trees could share their wisdom.

> I started to understand that there was some force of nature that allowed all living things to co-exist in a state of dynamic balance. . . . I then realized that, in a sense, trees do convey their wisdom to us through music; this is their voice. Music, as the sound of sacred, once-living substances is the voice of wisdom in nature. It is the vehicle by which we contact that force of nature that maintains a dynamic balance in both our inner and outer worlds. (Aigen, 1991, p. 92)

Carolyn Kenny's comments about the land and my experiences in Germany commit me to revisiting these thoughts and seeing them on a still more fundamental level. Trees spring from the earth, from the land itself. In this way, music is really the voice of the land, the way that earth, the earth, speaks to us. Much as our physical bodies hold the painful memories of our personal history, the land holds the history of a people. Music is also our conduit to our communal stories, particularly those painful memories which are so difficult to bring into consciousness.

The connections are complex but potent: My Jewish identity is connected to music; music comes from the land; the land holds history;

music tells the story of a land and its people; to be in a land is to feel its story through music. I sense that there is something for me to learn in this about myself and my relationship to music that will help me to be more authentic in my work as a researcher.

These thoughts bring me back to the Symposium in Düsseldorf.

I am on German soil for the first time. I once drove through Germany on my way from Denmark to France and did not once get out of my car, feeling like something terrible would happen to me if my feet touched the ground. Now I am lecturing on values, putting forth the essence of my cultural and personal identity in a place that represents something fearful within me, that holds the burden and the benefits of its history, as do all nations.

What is the music of the German soil and how does this relate to my decision to be here? There is a terrible ambivalence for me. On one hand, there is fear and a lifetime avoidance of exploring the feelings I have regarding Germany and my Jewishness; on the other, an affection for my colleagues in Germany and a deep appreciation for the opportunities for professional support presented by those who made the Symposium possible.

In a way, the only topic I could have spoken on was values. For me to be in Germany, on an unconscious level I had to bring the message of my tribe. It was a positive gesture that I could make in the light of our shared history. It was what I needed to do to further my own development and not remain tethered by the past.

In my talk I was implicitly saying: Is there enough of an overlap in our identities to build something together? Can my work be part of the healing of history? Can we connect through our values and beliefs, the things that make us who we are and that bind our communities? And, more personally, Can I see past my own fears and consider each person as an individual rather than solely through the lens of history?

There was also a darker side to my implicit message which has taken much discussion with colleagues and personal soul searching to realize. That is, by speaking about values, I was unconsciously attempting to establish myself as being in a morally superior position. It is possible that through the guise of discussing values I was also meeting an unconscious need to engage in moralizing. This is a painful realization, but one whose acknowledgement will make me a better researcher and methodologist because I will be less influenced by this unconscious need in my future writings and research activity.

These are the more individual questions. The larger questions concern how we reconcile our current self and the history of the group, tribe, or community to which we belong. My tribe has a history that I did not personally live through. I have been influenced by my group as well as isolated from a direct impact of one of its defining episodes. But the isolation exists only to an extent, and, as my self-exploration has shown me, history always affects us in the present.

We inherit the legacy of our group in all of its empowering and limiting aspects. If we deny this or fail to come to terms with it, it works in hidden and destructive ways, much the same as any unconscious conflict or prejudice. Conducting trustworthy, authentic, credible, valuable, reliable, or valid research—whatever qualifier we choose, the point is the same—necessitates that we come to terms with the aspects of our group membership, of our group history, that are active in our work as researchers.

What is it important to know? Although this is a good question to consider there is an equally important one that bears further examination: What is it important to say?

Perhaps this dialogue is interesting to you, perhaps you are helped in your development by it, and perhaps my earlier contribution to this volume is more intelligible or better contextualized for you now. Any and all of these outcomes would be worthwhile.

There is one other consideration. Maybe what we say publicly through our writings, talks, and correspondences serves as important a function for the writer as for the audience. As readers and listeners we are the ones doing the giving to those willing to share their work, their doubts, their uncertainties, and their growth processes, through professional forums. This thought is comforting to me and seems fitting given our identity as musicians and story listeners.

REFERENCES

Aigen, K. (1991). The voice of the forest: A conception of music for music therapy. *Music Therapy*, 10(1), 77-98.

Bruscia, K. E. (1996). Authenticity issues in qualitative research. In M. Langenberg, K. Aigen, & J. Frommer (Eds.), *Qualitative research in music therapy: Beginning dialogues*. Phoenixville, PA: Barcelona Publishers.

Kenny, C. B. (1996). The story of the field of play. In M. Langenberg, K. Aigen, & J. Frommer (Eds.), *Qualitative research in music therapy: Beginning dialogues*. Phoenixville, PA: Barcelona Publishers.

DIALOGUE 2

Qualitative Research in Music Therapy: New Contents, New Concepts, or Both?

Henk Smeijsters

INTRODUCTION

For me, one of the most important experiences in Düsseldorf was the discussion about criteria, rules, and guidelines in qualitative research. Most researchers argued that because qualitative research operates in a very different paradigm from quantitative research—one with its own conceptions regarding reality, how to achieve knowledge and generalization, and on the nature of causality and objectivity—it should have its own criteria for evaluation. Because I felt that, in essence, their way of doing research did not differ from mine, I asked myself why, without any cognitive dissonance, I still used the traditional criteria.

While preparing this Dialogue it became clear to me that I used traditional terms and concepts to describe new qualitative procedures. Other qualitative researchers in The Netherlands also do it that way. But I was not satisfied by telling myself that I was doing the right thing because other people in The Netherlands do the same.

So I wanted to ask myself if, as a qualitative researcher, perhaps I maintained preconscious quantitative thoughts. This Dialogue is an expression of my search into this matter and an explanation for why I want to use traditional terms when talking about new concepts.

CRITERIA FOR QUALITATIVE RESEARCH

Since Lincoln and Guba (1985) introduced the concept of trustworthiness, qualitative researchers seem to be astonished when concepts such as internal validity, external validity, reliability, and objectivity are used in qualitative research. In the conventional paradigm these four concepts were identified with procedures such as experimental design, representative sampling, test-retest replication, and the averaged intersubjective agreement. Because these procedures reflect different fundamental beliefs from the basic axioms of qualitative research the astonishment is understandable. If, as a qualitative researcher, you are convinced that there is no fragmentable reality and there are no simple causal relationships then using an experimental and control group to study the influence of an independent variable upon a dependent variable makes no sense. If you think context- and time-free statements are impossible you will argue that realities cannot be generalized, nor replicated, nor understood by a non-interacting inquirer. You will find sampling, repeated testing and the use of standardized scales useless. In qualitative research there are no variables, no effects, no control and experimental groups, and no measurements.

Lincoln and Guba rejected the concepts of internal validity, external validity, reliability, and objectivity because they believe that these concepts are inconsistent with the axioms and procedures of qualitative inquiry.

What seems to be forgotten, however, is that they also stress that for quantitative and qualitative researchers the same four methodological questions are appropriate (Lincoln & Guba, p. 218):

1) the truth of the findings of an inquiry for the respondents

2) the degree to which findings may have applicability in other contexts

3) whether the findings of an inquiry would be consistently repeated if the inquiry were replicated

4) the degree to which the findings stem from the characteristics of the respondents rather than from biases of the inquirer.

To me it seems possible that the concepts of internal validity, external validity, reliability, and objectivity can refer to these fundamental questions. The difficulty is that in quantitative research these concepts are defined in a reductionistic way and identified with the procedures of experimentation, sampling, replication and instrumentation. Lincoln and Guba use the concepts in exactly the same reductionistic and operationalized way quantitative researchers do.

In my opinion, however, these concepts can be still of value in qualitative research if they are described in another way and linked to procedures that fit the qualitative axioms.

Of course one may ask: Why hold to these concepts? I would like to answer this question with a personal argument, and arguments of parsimony and ease of communication. From my initial thinking about qualitative research it was clear to me that these concepts needed different contents, but I never believed in the inappropriateness of their use. I also believed that introducing new concepts that address the same questions raises barriers that hinder communication.

This is the same issue we are confronted with when communicating about music therapy in general: Should we completely develop a music therapy language of our own or should we integrate into our language concepts that can be understood by individuals from different disciplines? For example, do we need a theory of music therapy psychopathology and psychotherapy of our own or should we demonstrate that mental disorders as described by other disciplines are expressed through musical experiences? Music therapy is indicated because of musical processes that are able to trigger psychotherapeutic processes that can help to heal mental disorders (Smeijsters, 1993). In my opinion, we should link the language of music therapy with the language of other health professions.

The same holds true for qualitative research. We need a common ground that facilitates communication between quantitative and qualitative researchers. I am not saying that in essence these types of research are the same. They are "mutually exclusive ways of thinking about the world, and therefore cannot be integrated or combined within the same study" (Bruscia, 1996, p. 88). But when we respect the fundamental differences between the two approaches, then we also may ask if there are some shared methodological aspects of inquiry.

When we find these shared aspects, as Lincoln and Guba point out, we can ask if it would be fruitful to use a language which shows that indeed these questions are shared. What we can next consider is when and why a quantitative or a qualitative paradigm will be indicated to give answers to these questions. Whether a quantitative or qualitative approach should be used depends on the type of answers we want to give (the purpose of the study) and the attributes of the phenomena under study.

Of course this looks like some sort of a dilemma, because holding to conventional concepts includes the risk that the fundamental axioms of the qualitative paradigm are altered. However, I believe that using the conventional concepts in a new way can facilitate communication between researchers and also can respect the fundamental axioms of qualitative research.

Let us have a closer look at the new concepts introduced by Lincoln and Guba and try to understand what they mean.

Credibility (instead of internal validity) means testing if the reconstructions made by the researcher are credible to the constructors of the original multiple realities. Instead of causal links between fragments of reality the researcher describes complex mutual shapings, interrelationships between multiple aspects of reality. In this conception, everything influences everything else and each element interacts with all of the others. There is no directionality; phenomena simply happen.

The procedures to increase the probability of credible findings show that the researcher tries to prevent distortions, selectivity, and biases. The researcher wants to identify relevant characteristics, those things that really count. This interest resembles the interest of the experimental researcher who wants to know which variables really count.

Further, in qualitative research the researcher may investigate the process of enabling which means introducing elements in the context that do not cause changes, but make them possible (the word "element" is used by Lincoln and Guba). Even if there is no causal link it can be argued that there is some sort of an effect here.

An important goal of qualitative research is analysis, which can refer to the discovery of patterns, recurrencies, categories, types, regularities, or themes (Bruscia, 1995). Several papers that were presented at the Düsseldorf symposium fall into this category, such as Monologue 6 by Langenberg, Frommer & Langenbach and Monologue 5 by Amir.

When, as Bruscia discusses, the researcher looks at phenomena such as relations between nonverbal and musical events, changes in behavior after treatment, and the relations between verbal expressions of experiences and musical improvisations, there is no claim of linear causality. But this interest in connections of events, experiences, materials and personal characteristics, resembles the search for connections in quantitative research. Although the ideas about reality differ, a qualitative and quantitative researcher seem to share the same intention when looking for connections.

One can misunderstand the challenge presented by Ken Aigen (1996) in Monologue 1 of the present text when he says that he selects only those incidents for report that support his interpretations. There always needs to be a check whether the interpretations made by a researcher are grounded in the data and a check for the chain of evidence the researcher constructed. If there is not, the findings only reflect the personal view of the researcher and not the multiple perspectives of the participants.

Because qualitative researchers tend not to believe in the existence of an independent, external reality, the connections made by the researcher are not verified or falsified by their correspondence of lack of the same with reality. The connections are seen as reconstructions that have to make sense to those who made the constructions in the first place.

One could say the reconstructed patterns need to be sound, well-grounded, or valid as experienced by the participants. We could say also that they need to be internally valid which means sound for this unique context.

I would like to mention a seemingly paradoxical point. When notions of causality are rejected by qualitative researchers and, at the same time, credibility is assured by interaction with participants, then possibly the concept of causality needs to be introduced again because human beings—therapists and clients—construct their realities in terms of causal relationships.

Transferability (instead of external validity) addresses the question of how findings from one context can be applied in another context. There is no generalization of findings because a context is not considered a sample and every context is different. Only when there is a degree of similarity between sending and receiving context can the results of research be transferred. Therefore, a thick description of the sending context is needed, which is one of the primary tasks of the qualitative researcher. Although the basic axioms about reality and the procedures to reach applicability used by the qualitative researcher differ fundamentally from the quantitative procedures of sampling and generalization, for me, the concept of external validity stands for the well-groundedness of findings in another context.

Qualitative researchers do not strive to repeat a similar inquiry process in a given setting because of a belief that in social situations there is no stability. When thinking holistically there is no similar situation where one experience can be replicated in exactly the same way. Not only are human contexts constantly changing, the interaction between researcher and participants in qualitative research will never be the same, thus altering the design of a study. It is impossible to repeat a process which is more or less unique.

Instead of reliability, the concept of dependability was introduced to take into account these factors of instability. It seems to me that by using this new concept something is gained but something is lost too.

While it is not possible to repeat history it is still possible to repeat looking at it. The researcher can have different thoughts, feelings or images about the same experience at different times. Participants and observers, too, can have different thoughts, feelings and images about the same experience at different times. Research requires some sort of replication within and between human minds. The outcome is not presented as the truth but as a set of multiple perspectives. Thus, replication in qualitative research is possible, but it is not replication of the unique treatment but a replication of the descriptions of this uniqueness. There will emerge a never ending field of stories.

Qualitative researchers try to prevent distortions, selectivity and biases through prolonged engagement with the field of study. They also try to identify the most characteristic elements. Lincoln and Guba mention testing for misinformation. This testing happens by repeated observations and the use of multiple perspectives from different participants. For me, concepts such as intra-reliability and inter-reliability are more satisfying labels for these qualitative procedures.

Qualitative researchers argue there can be no objectivity because there is no objective reality and no truth. Realities are seen as subjectively constructed entities. Using the human instrument instead of standardized measuring instruments assures that in the reconstructions of the researcher the changing context, the meaning of this context, and the subjective perspectives of the participants will be included. No context laden with subjectivities can be understood without a researcher who from his/her own personal experiences tries to be open and empathic to these subjectivities.

Because objectivity in quantitative research was reduced to the average experience of a number of individuals, in qualitative research objectivity was replaced by confirmability. Lincoln and Guba conclude that the emphasis should not be on the investigator's characteristics but rather upon the characteristics of the data. But when they acknowledge that findings are grounded in the data, and that bias about the data is examined through peer debriefing and auditing, these procedures resemble the wish for objectivity in the traditional sense. The biasing of data descriptions by preconceived ideas, feelings, theories, and concepts by the researcher needs to be excluded.

RULES AND GUIDELINES IN QUALITATIVE RESEARCH

Because there are procedural rules in quantitative research, a researcher knows from the beginning of a study what to do and how to proceed. The hypothesis, the instrumentation, and the design are developed before research starts and there are no changes during the research process. In qualitative research, however, there is an emergent design which implies that there is no hypothesis, there are no measuring instruments, and there is no fixed design at the start. If there were, the essence of qualitative research would be lost because qualitative research is a process of interaction between inquirer and context of inquiry. If there is interaction there will be change in the method.

Qualitative researchers in music therapy often categorically hold to the rule that there are no rules in qualitative research. But again I would like to ask the following: What do we mean by a rule? How do we define the word "rule?" Is it, like the concepts of validity and reliability, defined in the conventional way?

I believe that the word "guideline"—which I introduced in my own qualitative research as outcome—would be better because a guideline can be used but one is not obligated to use it. If you interpret a rule as a prerequisite that assures that what you are doing is research and not clinical practice genuine application of the rule ensures the difference.

One of the dangers of the qualitative research paradigm is that sometimes everything seems to be research. As Bruscia (1996) points out, "research is not writing about one's clinical work, making up one's own theory, or sharing one's personal views" (p. 88). If these differences exist, we need rules to ascertain what is research and what is not. As with an inappropriate use of subjectivity, the negation of rules can also disguise poor scholarship.

In qualitative research there are rules too, and denying this is inauthentic as indicated by Bruscia (1996) in Monologue 4. Of course, not every technique or method to meet the criteria of internal validity (credibility), external validity (transferability), reliability (dependability), objectivity (confirmability) is used every time. Here the freedom to choose is expressed by the concept of a guideline. But whatever technique or method is used, we nevertheless need rules such as openness, interaction and dialectics to assure that we are doing qualitative research.

THE MUSIC THERAPIST AS A RESEARCHER

One of the justifications for interaction between researcher and participants is given by Lincoln and Guba (1985) who state that "meaningful research is impossible without the full understanding and cooperation of the respondents" (p. 105). With regard to therapy, Bruscia (1995) says that "qualitative research is enhanced when the researcher is the subject's therapist or when the researcher actively engages and interacts with the subject" (p. 75). This interaction between researcher and context is part of the qualitative paradigm. Because in therapy the therapist is the one who interacts closest with the client the roles of therapist and researcher can go together. In Monologue 1 in this text, Aigen combines the question of whether or not the therapist should be the researcher with the question of whether research should be done while treatment is in progress. I agree that combining treatment and research can be of benefit for the client.

When therapist and researcher are the same person we have a problem. This problem can be explained in terms of authenticity as Bruscia (1996) discusses in Monologue 4. Being a therapist is not the same as being a researcher. In therapy the therapist seeks insight for the client's sake, not for the sake of other clients. There can be inauthenticity when someone is not aware of his own perspective. If there can be this inauthenticity can it be handled methodologically?

I believe that it is very difficult to move between these two roles. It is much more easy and authentic when there are two persons, one who takes the stance of the therapist, another who takes the responsibility as a researcher. Then the problem of inauthenticity is minimized.

Bruscia's suggestion that the therapist/researcher is responsible for the authenticity of intent seems to be an insufficient criterion. We know that the awareness of our intent is often distorted. It is possible that a therapist can be as fully aware of this and can go into and out of these different roles. Yet it is a characteristic of research that these processes are more controlled and not only dependent on the therapist/researcher's self-monitoring.

SUMMARY OF CONCLUSIONS

Qualitative and quantitative research share some fundamental methodological concerns. The concepts that address these concerns can be the same but the procedures to implement the concepts can differ fundamentally because of different paradigms.

Qualitative researchers want to identify relevant characteristics, discover patterns, and study the process of enabling. The chain of evidence resulting from this should be internally valid as experienced by the participants in their unique context. It is also possible that the findings can be externally valid, which means that they may be of help in another context. Qualitative researchers use prolonged engagement, repeated descriptions, and multiple perspectives. Intra-reliability and inter-reliability prevent distortions, selectivity and biases. Peer debriefing and auditing check for inquirer biases and guarantee objectivity.

In qualitative research, some rules provide security that the activity is bona fide research rather than an extension of clinical work or theorizing. Rules also guarantee that the research is qualitative. Guidelines are methodological possibilities that can be used. Qualitative research can develop out of the unique context and unique interaction.

The music therapist can act as a researcher and it is important that the experience of the music therapist is part of the research. It is preferable to use a research team where the music therapist and researcher have separate responsibilities for reasons of authenticity.

REFERENCES

Aigen, K. (1996). The role of values in qualitative music. In M. Langenberg, K. Aigen & J. Frommer (Eds.), *Qualitative research in music therapy: Beginning dialogues*. Phoenixville, PA: Barcelona Publishers.

Bruscia, K.E. (1995). Differences between quantitative and qualitative research paradigms: Implications for music therapy. In B. Wheeler (Ed.), *Research in Music Therapy: Quantitative and Qualitative Perspectives*. Phoenixville, PA: Barcelona Publishers.

Bruscia, K. E. (1996). Authenticity issues in qualitative research. In M. Langenberg, K. Aigen & J. Frommer (Eds.), *Qualitative research in music therapy: Beginning dialogues*. Phoenixville, PA: Barcelona Publishers.

Guba, E. G. & Lincoln, Y. S. (1989). *Fourth generation evaluation.* Newbury Park, CA: Sage.

Kenny, C. B. (1996). The story of the field of play. In M. Langenberg, K. Aigen & J. Frommer (Eds.), *Qualitative research in music therapy: Beginning dialogues.* Phoenixville, PA: Barcelona Publishers.

Lincoln, Y.S. & Guba, E. G. (1985). Naturalistic inquiry. Newbury Park, CA: Sage.

Smeijsters, H. (1993). Music therapy and psychotherapy. *The Arts in Psychotherapy, 20,* 223-229.

DIALOGUE 3

Remembering What's Between the Lines

Carolyn Bereznak Kenny

My understanding of a dialogue is that it is two talking. Dialogues are always better when they are in person. When people are together they can engage in a free flowing exchange of ideas. The immediacy shapes the experience and thus the tone and texture of the encounter become informed by direct experience in the moment. People change in the talking. The result of this process is that we are responding to people instead of information.

I particularly like some of the characteristics of the Socratic approach to dialogues. In a professional community such as our Symposium group we serve dual roles as teacher and student to each other. In the Socratic method, the questions we pose to each other become more and more pointed to illuminate as yet undiscovered aspects of our thoughts, and to generate new ideas and previously hidden dimensions. We are midwives to each others' ideas.

Of course, responding on paper cannot replicate the experience of this oral tradition. We have not been roaming around in the town square together for years, mulling over the same and different thoughts. Our experiences in our relationships with colleagues are only a dim variation of the deep friendships which evolved in the Socratic community. However, I will respond to the monologues as "two talking."

In Düsseldorf we came together for a short period of time. It is merely an entree into a dialogical world. If the dialogues are to be productive there must be a developmental process over time. We must become more and more familiar with each other to build a community in which dialogue can deepen and enrich our work and our world.

It is a start.

To Mechtild, Jörg and Michael:

You might recall that when you sent me a copy of this work long before we arrived in Düsseldorff I was shocked at the similarities in our research. The image of the overlapping circles of therapist and client are exactly the same as the first part of the Field of Play. And the way you triangulated your study by including outside observers—the same as my study.

However, in Düsseldorf we never really discussed the similarities and differences in our research. We were too busy presenting our ideas and getting to know each other.

I was shocked once again, when I opened up the latest copy of *Music Therapy, 12*(1), the journal of the American Association for Music Therapy. A casual reader may ask: Is this not like the Field of Play? Do these people know each other? Are they in the same field? Do they live on the same planet?

The answer to all of these questions, of course, is yes. This is what happens when we design indigenous theoretical constructs and approaches to research. We are not connected.

But then again we are. Perhaps this is the area to explore. How did we come up with these similarities without prior knowledge of each other or of our work in music therapy, coming from two different cultures, two different languages. Does it say something about music therapy itself? Or does it say something about the spheres of influence which have helped to shape our thoughts, our approaches?

I imagine that you and I share a similarity in our familiarity with psychoanalytic thought and in particular object relations theory. D.W. Winnicott comes to mind. Is not his "transitional space" (more recently interpreted as "cultural space" by Murray Schwartz) similar to what we have conjured up? Also similar is our tendency to come up with mechanisms, such as the resonator function or double coding. I prefer to just say fields. But the question remains: Is it possible for any construction to maintain the necessary fluidity as we have in the sound? I question the components of the Field of Play for reducing, binding, constructing too much. I'm trying to keep this flexible and open but also to create a good foundation upon which to rest.

Where we begin to diverge is that my own ideas go on to articulate four fields: ritual, a particular state of consciousness, power, and creative process. I am very aware of the cultural influence of these particular fields. These are the longhouse for me. Walker Stogan, elder of the Musqueam Band, told me to go into the longhouse and listen. And I have been doing this ever since. I hear the sound in the longhouse all the time. It is part of my worldview.

We use both implicit and explicit interpretive structures. So we are both engaged in a hermeneutic process.

Where you go on and I do not is in my dogged persistence not to deconstruct the fields. I'm afraid of isolating variables because the territory is vast. What do we know, in fact, about how to deconstruct? Do we even want to deconstruct the person anymore, yet again, and to reconstruct based on our own image of health?

Your solution is a good one. You stay close to "quality" and "theme." This is soft. It also is still art. Indeed, it is hermeneutic, but it is more like art critique, leaning far to the left of quantitative or positivistic thought. It is idea-generating rather than idea-validating. You attempt to validate with the member checks, as I did.

A question for us is the following: Is deconstruction value-free? Obviously not. We have an agenda when we deconstruct. What is it?

To Dorit:

I was so happy to be sitting beside you in your presentation. I had watched your struggles to develop your work. I had participated in them. I had caused you to struggle as a consultant on your dissertation.

You and I have had many dialogues about this work. You presented it with clarity and purpose and because of this you helped me to define my own story.

My moments are still "beautiful." In this way I can maintain my enchantment with the senses, with the aesthetic experience.

There is a kind of intellectualism implied in the term "meaningful" within "significant moments." And I also see the value for clients and patients coming not always from the cognitive function but from the relationship between consciousness and the senses, and of course the experience of beauty from this joining.

"Meaning" remains a second order experience for me. Meaning is constructed in the mind.

You also frame your interpretations in time as "moments." My constructs are about "space." Space is primary for me.

In any case, when you and I discovered this moment business together, whatever we each name it, this was a precious moment to me.

This moment carried the deepest "meaning" and "beauty" of the concept of dialogue. This was a moment to remember. This moment continues.

To Ken B.:

In Düsseldorf, I watched you speak. Where were you going with all of this? You were trying to find yourself. Indeed, it did remind me of the paper you had presented at the New York Symposium in 1982. This had been another self-hermeneutic study. And here we are again, revisiting the self in the Music Therapy experience, countertransference, etc.

I was familiar with your work on the modes of consciousness because you had written it for our book: *Listening, Playing, Creating: Essays on the Power of Sound* (Kenny, 1995). And now you were taking the next steps.

In the paper on authenticity I heard a rain forest—a rich, chaotic, moist, earthy, busy exploration of Who am I? Who are we?

For me authenticity is a body sense. I don't have a mental construct for it. It is something inside my whole self. Maybe all those years of authentic movement did something to me.

I too was influenced at a ripe young age by the impeccable intellectualism of the Jesuit existentialists and haven't let go of their influence yet. I take heart in Sartre's dilemma. After all, in the Transcendence of Ego we hear the painful plea to stay in the body, stay in the life by his rejection of a transcendent philosophy. Sheepishly he admits his secret relationship to music in letters and interviews. He can't talk about music because it "means" too much to him, especially improvisation.

What do you think he would have thought of our experiences together in Düsseldorf?

In Music Therapy, I think the self-hermeneutic process must come before other interpretations if we are going to be authentic, especially as clinician-researchers. Our identification in the music is so subjective, often so deep, that the questions must be asked to reveal our underlying assumptions, our values, our beliefs, our spheres of influence, our imaginings and "constructions."

Where will you go from here?

To Henk:

You offer an important critical analysis of the difference between quantitative and qualitative research methods. What are the shortcomings of each? Which methods are appropriate for music therapy? How do we attend to validity and reliability?

I do not believe that we need to transfer the same validity and reliability checks across approaches. Each can have its own. I'm also not so sure that we must stay with the natural sciences. Why do this, other than our close association with medicine? We are not focusing on physical objects so much. The processes we are dealing with are not so predictable.

Cassell (1991), in *The Nature of Suffering and the Goals of Medicine*, says that the problem with doctors doing research is that they don't know how to tell a good story. So we have a bit of a reversal here. Cassell also attempts to introduce questions of value and aesthetics into medicine and medical research. His point is that practice and research in medicine is too often totally dissociated from the human condition of suffering.

I, too, am interested in the broader view of science, as is Ken Aigen. Couldn't we look at other approaches, other disciplines besides physical and natural sciences? We are not the only field asking this question.

Eisner (1981), in considering what he calls scientific and/or artistic approaches to research goes so far as to say that

> validity is the product of the persuasiveness of a personal vision; its utility is determined by the extent to which it informs. . . . Artistically oriented research acknowledges what already exists and instead of presenting a facade of objectivity, exploits the potential of selectivity and emphasis to say what needs saying as the investigator sees it. . . . It rejects the view that affect and cognition are independent spheres of human experience. (p. 5)

Eisner implies the art of rhetoric, but hopefully not Sophism. This is where your mention of the member check solution could be valuable, as long as we consider who the members are and their spheres of influence and possible vested interests. We could have intra-member checks, perhaps like the free phantasie variations. Then we could have inter-member checks, such as the check of panel members within the field. Then there could be extra-member checks, such as the ones employed by myself and Mechtild Langenberg in our studies.

From the field of linguistics, which bears many similarities to music and music therapy, Kramer proposes an evaluative model based on two criteria, point of view and innovation. According to Kramer, point of view means that a theory, for example, must be coherent and hermeneutically self-conscious. Its degree of innovation is made known by the way the author relates his position to previous positions taken in the field and establishes the uniqueness of his contribution to the phenomenon being studied. (Schumann, 1984)

Under Kramer's model of evaluation, it would be possible to argue that X's hypothesis has to be rejected because it is clearly less beautiful than Y's or X's position is ineffective because it unconsciously adopts the metaphor it seeks to discredit. Or perhaps X's position must be doubted because it forces me to deny my experience. (Schumann, 1984)

Certainly the entire area of hermeneutics is a rich exploratory ground for new research methodology in Music Therapy, as is heuristics. Both have been used here in contributions by Dorit Amir (1996); Mechtild Langenberg, Jorg Frommer, and Michael Langenbach (1996); Ken Bruscia (1996), Ken Aigen (1996), and myself (Kenny, 1996).

In hermeneutics we have the science of interpretation which is closer to art. Hermeneutics are ever-present anyway in Music Therapy, if we acknowledge the researcher as instrument, as suggested by Ken Aigen (1996) in his Monologue.

Once again we could use a variety of member checks, suggested by both yourself and Ken Aigen, and employed by Mechtild Langenberg and myself here. With an inter-member check, we may discover Kuhn's shared assumptions of a field. When we bring in "others," for extra-member checks we could address validity. In any case, looking at convergent and divergent ways of seeing and interpreting was immensely valuable to me in my study and significantly influenced not only my constructs but the subsequent model as well.

A question I have is how do we authentically operationalize variables? We have so many questions about knowledge here. What do we know really? From whence comes our knowing? If we are in any way limited in our knowing, how can we isolate variables ethically and with integrity? What is our agenda when we do isolate? How can we really claim to control? It's the category problem. I think we must also ask the question: What do we lose when we begin to isolate variables, as well as what do we gain? Maybe the stuff in between is the most important.

To Ken. A.:

In your study of values I see you attempting to encourage us to take seriously both the moral and aesthetic imperatives. By bringing up the complexity of the issue of values for both clinician/researcher and researcher we are taking Thomas Kuhn (1970) seriously now.

Overall, your article reminds me that we all have mixed feelings about subjectivity. We are caught in so many paradoxes in the Music Therapy experience. As clinicians our subjectivity is intensely valuable, at least equally as valuable as our objectivity. If it were not so prominent in our value system we would run the risk of dehumanizing our clients, of transferring categories from aesthetic experience to something else, of diminishing the creative process.

You bring up the importance of member checks. Is this, in fact, a way to monitor our subjectivity? Is it a way to check our realities, our perceptions, our effectiveness with clients?

I like the way you come to the question of what do we know anyway, through the values question. And I like the possibility of having both moral and aesthetic values.

How do we influence each other? This is another question to ask. If we are to establish new and better criteria for validity, this must be one of the questions we keep asking each other over and over again because we change.

Equally fascinating to me is the implied level of your work which could be formalized into an epistemology. It's about knowing and how we do it as Music Therapists. Perhaps this is even the entry point. What we know is in the music, in the sound. At least that's the way it is for me. Other things come second, including cognizing. The real "trustworthy" information is in the music. Do I always want to "decode" it? The answer is "no." But this poses a dilemma for research. How do we know if we don't think, then say? Maybe "knowing" is sometimes a sense.

To the Land, the Place, the People There:

I could not end without mentioning my experience, my dialogue with these. Sitting on the edge of the Rhine River with colleagues and friends was an intense experience for me. I only knew the Rhine as a youth, translating Caesar's Gallic Wars. To finally be on the Rhine close to my 50th year was an experience I'll never forget. To be in Germany was an experience I'll never forget. Prior to arriving I was full of many images of beauty and horror about Germany. This was the land of some of the poets and philosophers and musicians I hold most dear. It was also the place of some moments in history we would all like to forget. Germany and the United States have this in common, much blood on the soil. I found the land soft and green and lush, the people gentle and inviting.

Sometimes the chance encounters are the ones that linger on. I met a young man at one of our lunches. We began to discuss "the far right." How could it be? So soon, again. He offered me a German word meaning "the inner emptiness," something not to discuss on either side. I'll remember this too. I have remembered it many times already. I'm remembering it now.

REFERENCES

Aigen, K. (1996). The role of values in qualitative music. In M. Langenberg, K. Aigen & J. Frommer (Eds.), *Qualitative research in music therapy: Beginning dialogues*. Phoenixville, PA: Barcelona Publishers.

Amir, D. (1996). Experiencing music therapy: Meaningful moments in the music therapy experience. In M. Langenberg, K. Aigen & J. Frommer (Eds.), *Qualitative research in music therapy: Beginning dialogues*. Phoenixville, PA: Barcelona Publishers.

Bruscia, K. E. (1996). Authenticity issues in qualitative research. In M. Langenberg, K. Aigen & J. Frommer (Eds.), *Qualitative research in music therapy: Beginning dialogues*. Phoenixville, PA: Barcelona Publishers.

Cassell, E. J. (1991). *The nature of suffering and the goals of medicine*. Oxford: Oxford University Press.

Eisner, E.W. (1981). On the differences between scientific and artistic approaches to qualitative research. *Educational Researcher*, 5-9.

Kenny, C.B. (1995). *Listening, playing, creating: Essays on the power of sound*. Albany, NY: State University of New York Press.

Kenny, C. B. (1996). The story of the field of play. In M. Langenberg, K. Aigen & J. Frommer (Eds.), *Qualitative research in music therapy: Beginning dialogues*. Phoenixville, PA: Barcelona Publishers.

Kuhn, T. (1970). *The structure of scientific revolutions*, Second Edition, Enlarged. Chicago: University of Chicago Press.

Langenberg, M., Frommer, J. & Langenbach, M. (1996). Fusion and separation: Experiencing opposites in music, music therapy, and music therapy research. In M. Langenberg, K. Aigen & J. Frommer (Eds.), *Qualitative research in music therapy: Beginning dialogues*. Phoenixville, PA: Barcelona Publishers.

Sartre, J-P. (1937). *The transcendence of the ego*. New York: Farrar, Strauss and Giroux.

Schwartz, M. M. (1992). D.W. Winnicott's cultural space. *The Psychoanalytic Review*, 79.

Schumann, J. H. (1984). Art and science in second language acquisition research. In A. Guiora (Ed.), *An epistemology for the language sciences*. Detroit: Language Learning.

Lunch Talk:
Inner Emptiness, A German Problem

Gerd Rieger

When German therapists come together with therapists from other countries in a Symposium to talk about research, an outside observer can make some discoveries. He might ask himself the following: What is not discussed at the congress and stays hidden? What is rarely referred to but is present all the time? What depresses the mood and appears in the background? How are individual's perceptions of others affected by the recent headlines in the international press showing a great number of attacks against minorities in Germany?

While attending meetings with the participants of the *First International Symposium for Qualitative Research in Music Therapy* from Holland, Israel, Denmark, Finland, England, Italy, the USA, and Canada, I asked myself about the meaning of the results of National Socialism and its effects today. Do things such as war, capitulation, persecution, expulsion, the post-war period and Germany's partition have effects on a meeting of this kind?

In my work with evacuees and refugees from Poland and the former Soviet Bloc countries I am confronted time and time again with the consequences of war and the attempts of people to move beyond the trauma inflicted by it. The generation of people who were adults during the war deny the effects of that time and the following generation does not know the facts about the past. This made me curious about the ways in which the effects of national socialism are processed by individuals. I do experience a prohibition of speaking, a prohibition of memory, an enormous repression and at the same time an immense activism with which human beings want to reorganize their life in Germany.

The sensitivity of music therapists for their own history and culture keeps them open to things which may be repressed and split off in others. I wanted to consider how we minimize the importance of that which we partially deny and how we avoid putting unpleasant memories "on the stage again" (as does our parents' generation) as Germans in a meeting with therapists from other countries. Is this theme also a prohibited topic for music therapists? If so, I would find it regrettable, especially as we have to deal with the questions of migration, flight expulsion and the integration of foreigners in all countries.

The German Chancellor said that the guilt of Germans and participation at the events was not justified by the "mercy of the late birth." According to psychoanalysts there is no doubt that the following generation is also affected by past events in a special way. Possibly other participants in this Symposium also felt ambivalent about dealing with this resistance to memory.

During informal conversations and on the short walks to meals in Düsseldorf I felt that my colleagues wanted to hear from each other again, to exchange experience, to discuss directly this delicate theme. They wanted to relate this to their own lives, considering how Germans assimilate the things they deny or the things in which they involve themselves. A further consideration was the consequences this has for the following generations and how this part of history has a further effect on the patient's psyche.

In her book *National Socialism in the Second Generation: Psychoanalysis of Dependence Relationships* (1989), Anita Eckstaedt developed this theme for German therapists. She has created a portrait of the experience from diagnostic interviews and analyses. By the declaration of "hour zero" after the second world war, one has tried to deny the events without having to recognize or confess. The rebuilding in the post-war period diverted people's attention from a painful, critical examination of their own history. Thus, a prohibition to speak arose and the events were not allowed to be seen. Children adapted to the prohibition and developed an inner emptiness in response to it which was disordered and difficult to identify. It was a vague feeling of shallowness, confusing apathy, and depression. This inner emptiness possessed by the following generation could be a result of the outrageous effects and events not processed.

Eckstaedt has established the cause of this emptiness and disordered suffering as resulting from a dissatisfaction with the repression of memories engaged in by our parents' generation. If we, as German therapists, take part in the silence, a reconciliation with our parents' generation will not take place. The danger that outrageous abuses will return is a given. The wars in places such as Bosnia and in many countries of Africa remind us time and time again of these correlations and of their possible emotional consequences.

The interest in the discussion and the cautious questions of the foreign participants at this Symposium have encouraged me to continue the work on the question of the results of national socialism. It is not only a German phenomenon because force and aggression are international problems. The occasion of "Neo-Nazi" attacks and acts of violence against foreigners in united Germany makes these questions relevant for us as Germans.

Daedalus and the Labyrinth: A Mythical Research Fantasy

Kenneth E. Bruscia

Once upon a time in the Land of Enlightenment, there was a very wise king who cared very deeply about his people. And after many years of rule, he began to contemplate what legacy he would leave his kingdom. The king meditated and sought the advice of his council, asking each of them to ponder what would be of most value to the people.

Now each member of the council was in a different profession, and when the musician's turn came to give the king advice, she presented him with music that she had specially composed. The king was delighted that her message was embedded in her work and he listened very intently to each texture and strand of the music. In his rapture the king began to experience many puzzling images, each presenting very enigmatic questions. Then as the music came to a close, the king saw in his mind's eye a great labyrinth—the most fantastic one he had ever seen. Over its entrance was written: *Enter and seek, for herein lie the mysteries of life.*

The next day, it was clear to the king what he had to do. And so he summoned Daedalus, the cleverest of all architects in his kingdom, and said: "I charge you to build the largest and most challenging labyrinth in the world, for at its center I will place all the wisdom of my kingdom." Daedalus was honored to serve the king in this way, and worked for many decades to accomplish his charge. He designed and built each section of the labyrinth separately, destroying the blueprint of each as soon as it was completed. Thus, in the end, only Daedalus knew how to reach the center and only the King knew what mysteries would be stored there.

When the Great Labyrinth was completed, the King, very old by now, summoned all of his people, and announced: "Henceforward the gates of the Great Labyrinth shall open once each year for all those who have the courage of curiosity. If you persevere, wisely using all the gifts that I will provide to you, and if you reach the center of the labyrinth, you will find answers to the deepest mysteries of life.

The crowd began murmuring, excited yet unsettled by the king's challenge. After some time, individuals began to step forward, volunteering to be part of the first expedition. When a large enough group was formed, the king instructed Daedalus to distribute the special gifts he had prepared for them.

And Daedalus began: "With the king's generosity, I will present each of you a special gift that will help you on your journey. You may select whichever gift you wish, and upon doing so, you will gain the resources you need to accomplish your own personal mission; and at the same time, each gift will provide the entire expedition with an important clue to solving the riddle of the labyrinth. Be forewarned, however, no one gift or clue will be sufficient. You cannot succeed alone. You will only succeed as an expedition if you use all of the gifts that have been given to you."

"The first gift is this compass and book. With the compass, you will always know exactly where you are in relation to the center of the earth, and this in turn will help you to know in which direction you are headed within the labyrinth. In the book you will find maps of all the labyrinths that have ever been built—save this one. This will help you to understand the principle of the maze. Together they form the essential gift of truth. Be assured that no expedition into the labyrinth can go forward without some measure of it; but also beware, for truth is elusive indeed. Oft it is insufficient or irrelevant in its singularity. A truth is proven reliable only as it changes, and valid only as it is contradicted. And as soon as one captures it, one loses it; for in the certainty of knowing it, the untruth of it is concealed. Who shall accept and carry this essential but elusive gift on behalf of the expedition?"

And Henk came forward and said: "I shall take the compass and book. It shall be my responsibility to find where the truth lies, and where in its reliability and validity, it conceals and ignores what is missing. I will map out the labyrinth so that we know where the center of it is in relation to the world, for the mysteries of this Great Labyrinth must be accessible to all." The king was pleased, for he knew that Henk could approach truth with the gentleness of a blade of grass. And Daedalus passed this gift to Henk to use and to share with the others.

Daedalus continued: "The second gift is this exquisite gong. Whenever it is sounded, you will resonate with its every vibration. This will help you to feel and to understand what is in your heart, and in the hearts of each of your companions. While the gift of the gong is sensitivity, its challenge will be to recognize the differences between your sound and each of theirs. Be aware also that the gong can serve as a signal, for it can be heard throughout the entire labyrinth. Thus, if you should stray and become lost, upon sounding the gong, your companions will be able to find you. While the gong will always reveal where its player is, it may or may not tell you where the center of the labyrinth is. Who shall accept and carry this gift on behalf of the expedition?"

And Mechtild came forward with Jörg and Michael and said: "We shall take the gong, for with it, comes the responsibility to sound out how it feels to seek while also disclosing where each seeker is. If we find the center of the labyrinth, we will sound the gong to signal others into it." The king was pleased, as he had heard the empathy of their melodies, and the separateness of their timbres, and he sensed their aloneness together. And Daedalus passed this gift on to them to use and to share with the others.

"The third gift is this lovely butterfly. The beauty of its wings were inspiration for the labyrinth, and in their symmetry and balance, you will find the architectural principles used in its design. The gift of the butterfly is motivation, for the journey through the labyrinth and all the transformations that the seekers will undergo will be meaningless unless the beauties of the labyrinth and the journey itself are fully experienced. But beware, for the challenge will be its fragility. Notwithstanding the boldness of its transformation from the unsightly cocoon to its magnificent beauty as a butterfly, like motivation, the butterfly is easily destroyed: if you capture it, it will not survive; if you touch it, its wings will lose their colors; if you study it too closely, its lure will fade; and if you set it free, it may never return. Who shall accept and carry this delicate gift on behalf of the expedition?"

And Dorit came forward and said: "I shall take the butterfly, for with it, comes the responsibility of savoring each meaningful moment that we have in the labyrinth, whether that moment be one of confusion or discovery, disappointment or progress, perseverance or transformation, and regardless of whether any of us achieves the peak moment of reaching the center." The king was pleased, for he knew of Dorit's search for the beauty in life, and the meaning of all the changes she had seen in her world. And Daedalus passed the gift to her to use and share with the others.

He continued: "The fourth gift is this mirror. It reflects the brilliance of the sun, the subtle glow of the moon, and the shimmering of still water. When you extend its view, the mirror will reveal what is around the corner, and when you angle it with the sun, it will light up the darkest path, even transforming the light into heat. And whoever looks directly into it will see their own soul. The gift of the mirror is pure consciousness, and what it reflects as image is boundless. Paradoxically, the challenge of the mirror is to preserve your vision. For when it catches too much light, the mirror will blind you; and when it reveals without scrutiny, you will be tempted to close one eye; and when you look at it too closely, you will be unable to see what surrounds you; and when you reach out beyond its flat surface to the image inside it, you will lose where you are in the real world and plummet into the boundless space of eternity. Though viewers may deceive themselves through it, the mirror never lies—it is a double of who and what lies before it. It reveals who you are in all of your beauty and in all of your ugliness. Who shall accept and carry this gift on behalf of the expedition?"

And Kenneth from Bruscia came forward and said: "I shall take the mirror, for with it I will examine my own authenticity as a seeker, and by looking into my own soul and by sharing the mirror with my companions, I hope that the souls of other seekers will be likewise illuminated. This will enable us to bring our collective consciousness into the labyrinth, illuminating each path leading to the center." The king was pleased, as he knew that Kenneth learned much from being lost and losing himself. And Daedalus passed the gift to Kenneth to use and share with the others.

He continued: "The next gift is this bejeweled book. Inside it you will find all the laws governing our people, and on its cover you will see all the precious stones of our land. Together, they comprise the gift of values. The laws provide a moral code for what is considered right and wrong in the kingdom. The jewels on the cover match ones you will find on the walls of the labyrinth. The least valued stones will be found furthest from the center and the most valued ones will lead you closer to it. And upon following these clues, when you reach the center the jewels will reveal to you what has value within the center of the labyrinth and what does not. Like truth, the challenge of this gift is relevance. The laws of the kingdom may not be sufficient and relevant to what is right and wrong in the labyrinth; the precious stones of our land may or may not reflect values in the labyrinth. The person who bears this gift must constantly ask: By whose appraisal, and according to which standards shall we determine value? Who shall accept and carry this gift on behalf of the expedition?

And Kenneth from Aigen came forward and said: "I shall take this bejeweled book, for it will help me to discover my own values and the values of my companions. Owning our values will help us to understand the purpose of our mission, while also guiding our conduct in its pursuit and informing us of its accomplishment." The king was pleased for he saw that Kenneth understood the pain caused by injustice and judgment. And Daedalus passed this gift to Kenneth to use and share with the others.

He continued: "The next gift is the raven perched above. It cannot be caged or tied, it will only travel voluntarily, and it only goes with those persons who value its darkness." And Carolyn immediately stepped forward and said: "It will come with me. I know the Great Void, and have lived the energy of the raven."

And as the raven flew to her, Daedalus said: "This is the gift of magic. It is neither here nor there, its power is everywhere—and it moves of its own intent. It will not fly through any of the corridors in the labyrinth, though it is comfortable in their darkness. Instead, it flies freely above, in a field of play, circling ritually over the labyrinth, gaining an overview of it all. The raven can know the center only from above, it cannot travel very long on footpaths. Magically, it knows where you have been and where you are going, but it will not communicate it to you in ways that you either expect or desire. It flies alone in the sky, creating its own ceremony to heal the Earth."

And Carolyn replied: "I will be friend to the Raven, and work to understand its communications to us in the labyrinth. And if the Raven consents, I will also work to bring its magic and healing to all those who seek it during this journey." And the king was pleased that the Raven went to Carolyn, for he knew that Carolyn had mourned the loss of her ancestor's magic, and that she would use and share this gift with others in her own generation.

And Daedalus continued: "The king's final gift is this spool of golden thread. It is the gift of belonging, for it connects whatever it laces together. In its fragility, it imposes nothing—it merely hints of an attachment. It cannot hold you to it and it cannot force allegiance or affection. But when you are lost, and when you feel hopelessly alone, a pull on the thread will bring you back into the world of others. The challenge of the thread, however, is that though not easily forgotten when tied to it, it is easily broken. The thread will remind you to stay in touch with one another; it will keep you from forgetting or forsaking your gifts; and if you honor the thread, you will form life bonds with all those persons and things to which you become attached during your journey. Who shall accept and carry this gift on behalf of the expedition?"

And David came forward and said: "I will take this gift of thread, and with it, I will take responsibility for weaving relationships between and among seekers in the labyrinth and the gifts our king has bestowed upon us. And to serve as a reminder of whence we came, and to insure that we can find our way back home, I will tie one end of the thread to the entrance of the labyrinth." The king was pleased, as he knew that David valued a sense of belonging. And Daedalus passed the spool to David to use and share with the others.

After all of the gifts had been distributed the king stood over the expedition and blessed each of its members. "Go now and seek what the labyrinth of life will reveal to you. And whatever besets you upon your journey, remember above all else to cherish one another. For the labyrinth is not only a trial of seeking, it is a challenge of your individual humanity. If you cannot seek together, and love and respect the gifts of one another, then no matter how successful you are the labyrinth will be a very lonely and empty experience."

Bidding farewell to all, the expedition entered the Great Labyrinth, disappearing into its dark corridors. A reverent silence fell upon the crowd, and the King and Daedalus began their return home. Night fell and all the kingdom prayed for the success and safe return of the expedition.

But during the night the king suddenly fell seriously ill. In his wisdom, the king realized that it was his time to pass over, for the labyrinth had been given to him as his life's mission and now that it was complete the mystery of his own life was about to be fulfilled.

By the next morning, the king lay dying with Daedalus at his bedside. "Sire, tell me what your wishes are should the expedition into the labyrinth fail," Daedalus asked. And the king replied: "Those who enter the labyrinth may never find its center, but they shall never be lost, for in the Divine Plan, all those who have the courage to seek shall find the center of life and shall leave this world enlightened." And Daedalus pushed further: "But sire, what will they find there? What mysteries and wisdoms have you hidden in the labyrinth?" And the King replied: "They will find there what they already had here. For what each of them took as a gift was what they already had before going into the labyrinth, and yet, what they already had and brought with them is exactly what they still need to find. Be assured that what they discover will be unique to each of them, for each must make one's own journey to find one's own destiny. And as for the mysteries of life itself—I can say to you now what I have learned: Life has no mysteries, it is in the seeking that one's life is created and recreated for eternity."

And before the king's eyes closed for the last time, he made a final request of Daedalus. "Bury me near the entrance to the labyrinth, and tie the golden thread to my grave marker. As king, and guardian of the wisdom of this land, I have been unable to take my own journey through the Great Labyrinth, and though my body will forever lay outside of it, my soul longs to join the others and find its way home." His eyelids fell, and as the king drew his last breath an incredible beauty came over his face. At that moment, Daedalus realized that, in his death, the king had offered his final gift to the expedition. The gift this dear king would share with the others in the Great Labyrinth was the love he had in his soul. For Love was the most important of life's gifts that the king knew every seeker would need.

Issues in Qualitative Research: A Personal Journey

Dorit Amir

INTRODUCTION

The following is a personal narrative written in a qualitative manner. It describes my process after receiving the Monologues comprising the first section of this book from my colleagues. Margot Ely, my former teacher, writes that "there is a need to make more public the interplay between the emotional and the intellectual in ethnographic research, since this interplay is an essential ingredient" (Ely et al., 1991, p. 1). I want to share my journey with you so you can be part of my experience.

Upon receiving the Monologues from my colleagues at the Symposium, I became very excited. It felt like: Here we meet again! It gave me the feeling of being part of a shared community, a feeling I miss so much and really long for. I read all the papers and had a very personal experience with each one. Carolyn Kenny's (1996) work moved me very much. Throughout reading it I had a feeling of love and connection. The beauty of her story moved me, I could identify with its voice. It speaks to my heart. It suits my world view and my value system.

In Ken Aigen's (1996) Monologue I found myself smiling and agreeing with what he wrote. His article helped me organize my thoughts and ideas as a qualitative researcher in music therapy. It sounds familiar. We are both from the same "school of thought." I felt that things that I have known were put in a more clear manner for me. It left me with a good feeling.

While reading Ken Bruscia's (1996) Monologue I felt challenged. It stimulated my thinking. I had to struggle with the questions it brought up for me. I had difficulty with the precise manner and rules with which it was written.

Henk Smeijsters's (1996) Monologue left me frustrated. I found myself disagreeing with much of it. It is hard for me to read about qualitative research in positivistic language.

Mechtild Langenberg, Jörg Frommer and Michael Langenbach's (1996) Monologue excited me and I got very involved with the research process they presented: It stimulated me intellectually and I felt much passion and excitement about the new developments of the method and the research findings. I read my own paper (Amir, 1996) and realized that today I am in a different place from where I was when doing that research. There are things that I understand more fully today and therefore would do differently.

When I finished reading all the articles there was this voice in my head that said: "Oh! This is great! But what do you want to do with it? What are you going to write on? What do you want to focus on?" I really didn't know. I felt confused. I sat down and asked myself the following: What were the things that caught my attention in these Monologues? What were the issues which intrigued me as a researcher, as a professional, and as a human being?

I re-read all the Monologues and questions started to take shape. I wanted to find out why I felt so connected and moved in Carolyn Kenny's work. What were the specific ideas of Ken Aigen that I resonated with and in Henk Smeijsters's work that I did not feel at home with? What were the issues that challenged me in Ken Bruscia's Monologue? What excited me in the work of Mechtild Langenberg, Jörg Frommer and Michael Langenbach? And finally, What have I learned from reading my own Monologue?

While reading the Monologues for the third time, these questions became more specific. I would like to discuss three of them:

1) Why am I doing research and for whom?
2) What is the purpose of research?
3) What are the most important issues for me in doing and communicating research?

WHY AM I DOING RESEARCH AND FOR WHOM?

According to Kenneth Bruscia (1996), if I am authentic, I acknowledge that I am doing research for:

1) Me and you as scholars/therapists;
2) Future clients of my own and those of other therapists;

3) When appropriate, the clients who provided the original data.

This list stimulated me to think hard about this issue and to question myself: Why am I doing research? What is my motivation to do research? For whom am I doing it? Who is going to benefit from it? I have to admit that the first person that I am doing research for is me. Me, as a researcher, as a clinician, as a supervisor, as a teacher and as a human being. I want to increase my knowledge. I want to better understand the work I and my colleagues do. "Many of us are motivated to do research precisely because we want to find out more about clinical practice, often our own", says Aigen (1996, p. 15).

I want to share my understanding with other colleagues both within and outside my field so I can get feedback and learn more about what I did. It is important to me to share my work so other professionals can get to know me better. I want to benefit from my research so I can be a better researcher, clinician, supervisor, teacher and human being. I want to grow professionally and personally.

For me, qualitative research is not only a method of inquiry, it is a way of life. It is how I view the world and is connected to my values and beliefs. Carolyn Kenny (1996) gives a very authentic answer to this question: "Why am I doing this? The answer was clear. For the Beauty" (p. 57). Her motivation for doing her research and telling her story was to find a way of honoring the experience she had with her client "by telling the truth" (p. 58). This is not an objective, ultimate truth. It is a personal truth and in this way truth and meaning are the same.

Second in priority, I am doing research for the client(s) and therapists who I study. In qualitative research, one of the tools we use as researchers to gather data is the intensive interview. Clients in music therapy can benefit directly by being interviewed. They have an opportunity to tell their story, their personal truth. They can gain new insight into the experience while talking about it in the form of an interview. Through seeing the experience from the distance of an interview they can gain clarity on issues they had worked on. In the study discussed in my Monologue (Amir, 1992) it was important for me to hear what clients in music therapy had to say about their experience so I could be a voice for them.

Often, as therapists we are the ones who claim to know more and interpret our clients' inner experiences, sometimes without asking them. In my study, some of the participants (clients and therapists) gained new insights into their experience while being interviewed. Most of them commented that they enjoyed talking so openly about their experiences in music therapy, something that they do not normally do. Aigen (1996) thinks that a client could benefit from the increased level of attention as his/her therapist gains more insight into the client's process. Clients also, continues Aigen, might benefit from the feeling of being important and having a direct impact on the profession. Their participation in qualitative research studies, concludes Aigen, gives them a voice that they do not have in any other place. One of the considerations that Aigen had while doing his research was that "the research should have relevance for the therapists in the study, and, in some way, help them to better understand and help their clients" (p.18) Indeed, the interviews he did with the therapists of the group he researched in *Here We Are in Music* (Aigen, in press) stimulated them to see the group in different ways and to better understand their roles in the group.

Third on my list are music therapists in general. Indeed, I want to contribute to the body of knowledge and as Bruscia writes, "to gain insight for the scholarly community" (1996, p. 83). At the end of many research studies we see recommendations for further research and suggestions on how other researchers can continue to try, check, develop, and expand methods, approaches, procedures and guidelines, and, in this way, generate more findings and enlarge the communal body of knowledge.

Last on my list is the larger community of professionals in related therapies, working in various positions, such as clinicians, educators, and administrators. Most people external to the profession of music therapy want evidence that it works. They want to know what works and what does not work, presented in a clear and precise manner. They want to know about causal relationships in therapy and to read the bottom line. Most of the professionals in music therapy and in related disciplines think positivistically. Only by doing research in a way that is congruent with the experience in music therapy, research that speaks my truth as well as that of my clients, can we eventually bring a change of perception in the larger scholarly community.

WHAT IS THE PURPOSE OF RESEARCH?

The purpose of research is to gain knowledge, to gain insights into the known and unknown aspects of the phenomenon being researched, to get to the essence of the phenomenon, and to let it speak to me so I can understand its meaning. The question is, what kind of knowledge are we talking about? I do not see the purpose of research as being to prove what does and does not work in therapy. I do not see the purpose of research as achieving a better understanding of cause and effect relationships because I see reality as multiple, changing and transactional, as a web, as "fields within fields within fields" (Wilber, 1983, p.83). Every human being is a unique person who is developing and changing from moment to moment. What works with one client in one moment in time may not be effective for another client or for the same client in another moment.

I also do not believe in seeking to establish causal relationships in music therapy. In the multiple realities view there is no linear link between cause and effect. For me, the aim of research is to gain knowledge about human experiences in the context of music therapy.

This is one of the reasons I became so interested in the research study of Langenberg, Frommer, & Langenbach (1996). In doing their research on musical improvisations produced in music therapy, they were interested in "understanding the feelings and thoughts involved in the interpersonal encounter that is the basis of improvisation" (p. 157). In order to grasp the interaction between therapist and client in the music, they looked for methods appropriate to the experience, "methods that do justice to the holistic character of this therapy, a process with its own structures and meanings" (p. 134).

Every research study has its own specific purpose that is illustrated by its title and research questions. Henk Smeijsters (1996), for example, explains that one purpose of research is to study the process of change in psychotherapy: "During the treatment small changes take place and the study of these changes offers insight about when and how effects occur and what triggers them" (pp. 36-37). I would like to conclude this section of the Dialogue by quoting what Carolyn Kenny (1996, p. 65) says in her Monologue: "After all, what is research for, if not to learn and to understand, to improve and to change, to grow?"

WHAT ARE THE MOST IMPORTANT ISSUES FOR ME IN DOING AND COMMUNICATING RESEARCH?

I realized that there are three things involved for me: being authentic in conducting and reporting the findings of a research study; finding new language that suits the music therapy experience; and, building a shared research community. Because I talk about authenticity throughout my paper, and it has to do with all the aspects that I mention here, I do not write about authenticity as a separate section.

Finding New Language

For me, one of the main purposes of doing research in music therapy is to find language that is congruent with the experience. I have a need to find out what forms and contents of language can authentically describe the music therapy experience, including its inherent, hidden qualities. How can we best describe music that is the essential and unique element in our work?

In her Monologue, Carolyn Kenny (1996) presents her experience in music therapy as a story. The way she writes moves me. It speaks to me. I get so involved in the story that it comes to life in my inner world: I can hear the sounds, I can see the whole scene, I can feel the drama. This form of writing is open, dynamic, moving, developing, allowing for beauty, love, intuition and wisdom. It is exactly like some of our music therapy sessions, or supervision sessions, or teaching a class of students, or improvising alone or together, or reading a book, or having a conversation with a friend. When we feel moved, we feel we create something, we feel it is meaningful and it has beauty. It speaks the truth for us and perhaps for the others involved too. When does it happen? When we are committed, when we are fully in the here and now and completely immersed in the present, when we know in our hearts that this is the truth, our truth.

In the research reported in Monologue 6, Mechtild Langenberg, Jörg Frommer and Michael Langenbach (1996) organize their data according to "qualities" and find motifs that describe the experience. They find that "a verbal transformation (of music therapy sessions) offers the option to look at the full range of possible associations with music, such as connecting music with some vivid images, with emotional states or with particular events in people's lives" (p. 151). However, because music is more than its verbal translation, they add a musico-graphical perspective so one can see tensions, opposites and other things. This is exciting! The combination of two forms of new language, verbal and musico-graphical, gives me the ability to grasp the session and understand the structures and meanings of it in a holistic way.

Henk Smeijsters (1996) says that "concepts develop while observing processes in a natural situation. The procedure of formulating concepts is based on 'openness' to and feedback from the data" (p. 36). Being open to data encourages me, as the researcher, to develop new language and concepts that will be faithful to the participants' experiences without imposing pre-existing concepts upon the data that is taken from natural experience. Henk disagrees and argues that "in qualitative research the old concepts still can be used if their contents become accommodated to the characteristics of qualitative research" (p. 39). When he talks about the procedure of reassuring accuracy of the findings, he is using the language of positivistic research, including concepts such as reliability and validity.

I find it difficult to use this language. For me, these concepts belong to a different paradigm and they are not congruent with qualitative work. In this matter, I like the terms "trustworthiness" (Lincoln & Guba, 1985) and "authenticity criteria" (Guba & Lincoln, 1989). We need to be honest and to speak the truth. The beautiful thing about qualitative research is that it allows for ambiguity. It respects the uncertain. It cannot be precise in a positivistic manner—we do not know exactly what is going to happen in the research process, as is the case in our clinical work and in life. The research questions and focus are shaped throughout the process. No one begins research without questions, but these can be very broad and shape themselves or even change as the process proceeds. If you have a focus and stick to it right from the beginning, you might not be open to the lived experiences of the research participants. You might not be listening to what is really going on there, thus missing the authentic experience and not allowing the focus to change accordingly.

Building a Community

All of us write about the need for a community of researchers. Kenneth Aigen (1996) talks about the communal identity of a group of people who share certain values, beliefs and forms of knowledge and Kenneth Bruscia (1996) calls it a scholarly community. Carolyn Kenny talks about the need for a community: "Together we will construct a reality, a world . . . which makes sense, given our shared experience in the field" (1996, p. 55).

What do we need to do in order to build a community? First, we need to establish our communal identity. We need to identify ourselves as music therapists-qualitative researchers. I found one of the means for building this community in Carolyn Kenny's Monologue:

> We can support and challenge each other by screening out the last remnants of the positivistic view, particularly language, concepts, assumptions, values, accommodations of various kinds to the old approach, proving, cause and effect. . . . When we claim our place, there can be a more productive dialogue amongst ourselves and with others who hold different world views. (Kenny, 1996, pp. 59-60)

Second, we need to get to know each other. We need to listen to each other in a qualitative way: to make the familiar unfamiliar and to make the unfamiliar familiar. This is not an easy task. It means accepting our colleagues as they are. To respect the uniqueness of each one and to embrace not only the commonalities but also the differences among us. "It is important for us to support each other," says Aigen (1996, p. 13). Only when we dialogue, share and compare can we help each other grow and have a stronger sense of personal and professional identity. This is the way to build a communal identity. As a community we can present ourselves to the others in a stronger fashion.

I would like to end this personal narrative by sharing with you something about myself, where I come from, and talk about building a shared community in a different, broader perspective. I was born in Israel and have lived there with a very beautiful Jewish tradition along with the pain of living day to day with the Israeli-Arab conflict. Because of this, it is my dream to create such a community between Israeli and Arab people, a community where people of both sides study and gain knowledge of each other qualitatively, learning to respect each other's values and opinions, learning to accept each other and to listen to and create dialogue with each other. This is the only way to bring out the beauty and wisdom that both societies have. This is peace.

REFERENCES

Aigen, K. (1996). The role of values in qualitative music. In M. Langenberg, K. Aigen & J. Frommer (Eds.), *Qualitative research in music therapy: Beginning dialogues.* Phoenixville, PA: Barcelona Publishers.

Aigen, K. (in press). *Here we are in music: One year with an adolescent, creative music therapy group.* Nordoff-Robbins Music Therapy Monograph Series #2.

Amir, D. (1992). *Awakening and expanding the self: Meaningful moments in the music therapy process as experienced and described by music therapists and music therapy clients.* Doctoral Dissertation, New York University. UMI Order # 9237730.

Amir, D. (1996). Experiencing music therapy: Meaningful moments in the music therapy experience. In M. Langenberg, K. Aigen & J. Frommer (Eds.), *Qualitative research in music therapy: Beginning dialogues.* Phoenixville, PA: Barcelona Publishers.

Bruscia, K. E. (1996). Authenticity issues in qualitative research. In M. Langenberg, K. Aigen & J. Frommer (Eds.), *Qualitative research in music therapy: Beginning dialogues.* Phoenixville, PA: Barcelona Publishers.

Ely, M., Anzul, M., Friedman, T., Garner, D., & Steinmetz, A. M. (1991). *Doing qualitative research: Circles within circles.* New York: The Falmer Press.

Guba, E. G. & Lincoln, Y. S. (1989). *Fourth generation evaluation.* Newbury Park, CA: Sage.

Kenny, C. B. (1996). The story of the field of play. In M. Langenberg, K. Aigen & J. Frommer (Eds.), *Qualitative research in music therapy: Beginning dialogues.* Phoenixville, PA: Barcelona Publishers.

Langenberg, M., Frommer, J. & Langenbach, M. (1996). Fusion and separation: Experiencing opposites in music, music therapy, and music therapy research. In M. Langenberg, K. Aigen & J. Frommer (Eds.), *Qualitative research in music therapy: Beginning dialogues*. Phoenixville, PA: Barcelona Publishers.

Lincoln, Y. S. & Guba, E. G. (1985). *Naturalistic inquiry*. Beverly Hills, CA: Sage.

Smeijsters, H. (1996). Qualitative single-case research in practice: a necessary, reliable, and valid alternative for music therapy research. In M. Langenberg, K. Aigen & J. Frommer (Eds.), *Qualitative research in music therapy: Beginning Dialogues*. Phoenixville, PA: Barcelona Publishers.

Wilber, K. (1983). *Eye to eye: The quest for the new paradigm*. New York: Shambhala.

Interpretation and Epistemology in Music Therapy
or
How to Deal with Competing Claims of Knowledge

Even Ruud

It is an underlying assumption among most of the contributors to the present collection that the aim of qualitative research in music therapy is not to reach some kind of truth in the sense of describing a single reality. There is also an assumption that a particular method does not guarantee that the results can be compared with some pre-set standard of truth. Or, as Ken Aigen says in his opening Monologue:

> Method is neither a guarantor nor an arbiter of truth. Because so much of qualitative research is dependent upon the skills, personal qualities, and insight of the researcher, it is possible that a given method could be meticulously followed and still not produce valuable or trustworthy findings. (1996, p. 24)

Instead, qualitative research acknowledges the existence of multiple realities, "that truth and reality exist in the form of multiple, intangible mental constructions" (Bruscia, 1996, p. 88), and that the best we can accomplish is to reach a better understanding of the particular reality I am involved in or share in some areas with a particular client. Does this mean, then, that qualitative research is not concerned with possible competing claims of knowledge? Or, how are various aspects of validity dealt with in the present collection of papers?

If we take a closer look at the Monologues we will find that there are approaches which live up to this ideal of relative truth and reports which try to obtain some kind of validity in the traditional sense. Henk

Smeijsters (1996), for instance, although he recognizes the importance of qualitative designs in music therapy research, finds it important, not to give up "the accepted criteria for sound scientific research" (p. 35). Smeijsters argues that we need criteria for validity, and, thus, sees the problem of validity as a methodological one. It is a problem to be solved within his empirical or positivist epistemology. It could be questioned, however, if the problem of conflicting claims of knowledge is a methodological one or if it belongs to the epistemological domain. If the latter is the case, we shall have to deal with different epistemologies pertaining to various methodological approaches. It is not, then, a question of taking traditional methodological precautions to ensure validity.

In the positivist paradigm, we find the correspondence theory of truth which is based on how well data correspond with reality. As opposed to this, data in qualitative research are considered to be in some way constructed. Because there is no way of knowing reality direct-ly—knowledge is mediated through language and perception—the qualita-tive (or hermeneutic) effort aims at revealing the meaning or significance of data. This is in accordance with the broader interpretative background, the hermeneutic concept of truth, or what is sometimes called the coherence theory of truth. The coherence criterion refers to the unity, consistency and internal logic of a statement (see Kvale 1989). Thus, Aigen (1996), when he talks about accuracy, does not mean "correspon-dence" but "appropriate [metaphoric] representation" (p. 25).

There is also a third concept of truth prevailing in contemporary theory of science, i.e. the pragmatic point of view, which is concerned about truth being measured against its practical consequences, its usefulness (see Alvesson and Skoeldberg, 1994).

The triangle in Figure 1 represents the various positions.

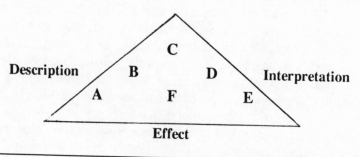

Figure 1. Positions regarding the nature of "truth" in science.

This model could help us to understand some of the paradigms dominating different schools of research in today's music therapy. Let us first take a look at the traditional conception of science. If research in music therapy was completely identified as outcome research, we could apply a pragmatic criterion to evaluate whether the knowledge we have produced is true. This is recognized in the model as position F. Behavioral studies, for example, are concerned with the contingent use of music, that is with its effect upon behavior, not its meaning for the patient.

The problem with such a position is that it would tell us nothing about the processes leading towards change in behavior nor would it describe how music is an important facilitator in the process. Moving leftward in our model, we will find Researcher A who not only will try to account for the changes in the behavior of the client, but will have made a description, or an operational definition of the music being used or the behavior involved. This is often done within the paradigm of empirical epistemology by applying concepts from physics or acoustics in order to obtain correct data or intersubjectively shared statements. Therapist A, then, finds herself in a descriptive-pragmatic mode where the question of the significance of music is downplayed and where descriptions (of music or behavior) are close to empirical data. This is also a practice where theory building has less importance than theory corroboration and verification. (In this sense the *Journal of Music Therapy,* published by the National Association for Music Therapy in the USA, is the most recognized chronicle of the music therapy verification-proletariat.)

Position B is assumed by the positivist researcher most concerned with describing data. In research, the analysis of music is put into focus. This will lead to a detailed description of the musical parameters according to some system of analysis. In some of these systems, analysis often starts from this level, either close to the score, transcription or (phenomenological) experience. Some close readings of the music done by phenomenologists would belong in the area between B and C, depending upon the recognition of their own preunderstanding (Husserl-Heidegger).

It is interesting to see how phenomenology is coming close to a positivist standard of truth when insisting upon describing the essence of a phenomenon. Thus, in her Monologue, Carolyn Kenny (1996) brings herself out of such a position by insisting upon the fictional and narrative character of her description of the pure essence. Of course, Kenny also distances herself from the positivist epistemology by not claiming any universal truth in her statement that "we cannot assume that the eidos is universal" (1996, p. 62). She insists, however, upon the discovery of the essence in her story and this is how her project becomes paradoxical, both essence and story. But in order not to stay in her paradox Carolyn Kenny tries to demonstrate narrative coherence in the presentation of her theoretical narrative.

The analyst taking position C would try to take a stand at which the investigation of the phenomenon reveals the nature of the phenomenon, in the sense of saying something about its significance. Although not fully recognizing that this meaning is a construct, or taking into focus the full account of a deeper cultural or biographic meaning, analysis would tend to stay close to the structure of music or the supposed "natural categories" evolving from the close investigation of the experiences of the patient.

A researcher in position D removes herself from the idea of the possibility of describing music or the experience of the patient as it is, or the true experience of the patient. There is always a deeper underlying theme, hermeneutic interpretation, or a significance which may be interpreted. We can clearly see this in Monologue 6 by Langenberg, Frommer, & Langenbach (1996) and in Monologue 5 by Dorit Amir (1996) in which she states: "I wanted to find out more about the meaning of the experience of music therapy for those who are involved as therapists and clients" (p. 110). Although Amir explicitly describes the process which leads to her categories, it could be discussed to what extent her categories are constructed. Both Langenberg, Frommer & Langenbach and Amir seem to be faithful to the orthodox tenets of grounded theory, thus focusing the empirical nature of their categories. This empiricist turn is supported by Amir's list of credibility measures: intensive contact with subjects, triangulation, peer debriefing, negative case analysis and member checks, some of which we have recognized in Henk Smeijsters' (1996) Monologue as constituting the scientific single case study. Thus, Amir's hermeneutic approach to the "meaning behind" is somewhat inflected by the empiricist epistemology. The same may be stated about the Langenberg, Frommer, & Langenbach study, which also tries to strengthen aspects of validity by using a panel of interpreters.

In all of the Monologues there seems to be less of the the postmodern turn in qualitative research, where the researcher may even find the text (music, experience) irrelevant as an authentic expression informing us about the inner life of the patient, taking into consideration only the text as being produced within the context of other texts. That is, music improvised, for instance, is not understood with reference to some underlying structure of the music or to the biography of the patient but to the musical code developed throughout the previous sessions. Kenneth Bruscia (1996), for instance, is not openly advocating the discursive or narrative character of his knowledge in Monologue 4; he is more concerned about the credibility of his approach. In this elaborate and convincing discussion of authenticity the question of possibly competing claims of knowledge has become a question of how to secure the trustworthiness of knowledge. This approach introduces rhetorics as an important vehicle in the communication and constitution of knowledge. Perhaps Bruscia would rather move towards position E where interpretation will take into its focus its meaning and the clinical signification of music therapy.

Moving towards position E would also allow the narrative and rhetorical character of our knowledge to partake in the important task of theory building in our field. At the same time we would have some necessary feedback from the larger intersubjective community of therapists about the reality of our thoughts and actions.

REFERENCES

Aigen, K. (1996). The role of values in qualitative music. In M. Langenberg, K. Aigen & J. Frommer (Eds.), *Qualitative research in music therapy: Beginning dialogues.* Phoenixville, PA: Barcelona Publishers.

Alvesson, M. & Skoeldberg, K. (1994). *Tolkning och reflektion. Vetenskapsfilosofi och kvalitativ metod.* Lund: Studentlitteratur.

Amir, D. (1996). Experiencing music therapy: Meaningful moments in the music therapy experience. In M. Langenberg, K. Aigen & J. Frommer (Eds.), *Qualitative research in music therapy: Beginning dialogues.* Phoenixville, PA: Barcelona Publishers.

Bruscia, K. E. (1996). Authenticity issues in qualitative research. In M. Langenberg, K. Aigen & J. Frommer (Eds.), *Qualitative research in music therapy: Beginning dialogues*. Phoenixville, PA: Barcelona Publishers.

Kenny, C. B. (1996). The story of the field of play. In M. Langenberg, K. Aigen & J. Frommer (Eds.), *Qualitative research in music therapy: Beginning dialogues*. Phoenixville, PA: Barcelona Publishers.

Kvale, S. (1989). To validate is to question. In S. Kvale (Ed.), *Issues of validity in qualitative research*. Lund: Studentlitteratur.

Langenberg, M., Frommer, J. & Langenbach, M. (1996). Fusion and separation: Experiencing opposites in music, music therapy, and music therapy research. In M. Langenberg, K. Aigen & J. Frommer (Eds.), *Qualitative research in music therapy: Beginning dialogues*. Phoenixville, PA: Barcelona Publishers.

Smeijsters, H. (1996). Qualitative single-case research in practice: A necessary, reliable, and valid alternative for music therapy research. In M. Langenberg, K. Aigen & J. Frommer (Eds.), *Qualitative research in music therapy: Beginning dialogues*. Phoenixville, PA: Barcelona Publishers.

DIALOGUE 8

Translations

Jutta Baur-Morlok

Some of the Monologues in this collection are concerned with the attempt to grasp what happens in music therapy, first in order to learn from it and then to make it comprehensible for further scientific processing and evaluation. This inspired me to think about the role of translation in the different therapeutic techniques.

As a non-verbal therapy, music therapy offers the advantage of a complementary medium to verbal language in which one's internal world can be expressed and communicated to others. On one hand, an essential element of music therapy is to provide a pure cathartic experience which one goes through in an emotional manner operating on the level of primary process. On the other hand, there is an exchange between two levels of experience, one of music and the one of language. What has been perceived on one level can been translated and transposed into the other level. This works in both directions: from the medium of music to verbal language and from verbal language to music. Both of these possible directions appear in the terms as a reference point: in the term "music therapy" the naming medium is music, whereas in the term "non-verbal therapy" it is language which gives the name.

Because they use a non-verbal technique, some music therapists claim to have special access to the immediate experiences that are pre-linguistic and barely organized according to secondary processes. It is thus possible to receive and to reproduce the emotional level and to catch regressive processes in a rather unreflected and uncensored way. And this may in fact be in the service of the ego and may thus lead to further secondary process and integration. In order to reach enduring changes, the therapeutic experience must finally go through affective involvement and must reach this level again and again. It is only here that we can achieve changes and integration of the internal representations. This is typical of all non-verbal therapies.

It only appears, however, as if something unique to non-verbal therapies is taking place; in fact, this is true for all therapies which are psychotherapies in a strict sense, i.e., focused on changing internal personality structures. This capacity also applies to the therapies that exclusively rely on the medium of verbal language and this is valid also for psychoanalysis. Even as concerns this therapeutic technique—in a bit short-sighted point of view—we often believe that what only matters is insight.

Psychoanalysis has now established a language to make this distinction understandable. There is, for example, the term the "therapeutic split of the ego" which facilitates the understanding and perception of an understanding of what one experiences, says, or does, during the analytic session. From a sociological point of view, this means the ability to change perspective, not between ego and alter-ego, but between different levels of organization, or, in other words, taking a meta-perspective. All cathartic therapies, however, do without focussing and taking advantage of this change of levels. This might be the case in cathartic non-verbal music therapy and in verbal hypnosis therapy, for example.

In psychoanalytic treatment which only allows verbal expression, it is much more difficult to fix that level on which patient and therapist are at a given moment. Everything is language, there is no helpful distinction between two clearly separated media where one can serve as meta-language for the other, and where, moreover, we should have a temporal and spatial separation in the therapeutic setting itself. Psychoanalysts must ask themselves and the patient again and again which of different levels is referred to in a given situation, which shall be put in the foreground, and how different levels can be brought together in one statement in the present.

But the point here is not that analysis is required from the very begin-ning, that is only step number two. The point is acting, even if this acting only means acting by talking, but often we also have (verbal and/or nonverbal) symbolic interactions. Taking the meta-perspective means changing the point of reference, and just by doing this we can create a new level. Thus, in psychoanalysis, we also have these two fields that cannot be distinguished so very plainly as in non-verbal therapies. These are privileged having established the distinction into two different media in the setting itself. Thus, music therapy, for example, distinguishes between discussing and finding a theme, playing an impro-visation and discussing again. Guided Affective Imagery also has preliminary discussion and finding a theme, then imagery itself and dis-cussion afterwards.

In psychoanalysis we also have fields that can be distinguished more easily, for instance when a dream is reported. The dream report is something that is firmly outlined and that can be distinguished from talking about the dream. The dream report then is the "story," it is the (mutual) work, often specially emphasized in the language with a special opening: "I now would like to tell you a dream . . . ". In the dream report, however, the distinction between the levels of telling and commenting can become obscured and change quickly. It is as if in music therapy a patient commented while playing an improvisation and made accompanying and explanatory comments as well.

The term "free association" also indicates a change into another medium, even if this is language, too. This weighty term, however, suggests to a greater extent what might be distinguished separately than what one typically finds in analytic treatment.

The distinction between working alliance and transference is also an attempt to distinguish between both of these levels; a separation also criticized as being too artificial because it is said only to pretend that there are different levels "in reality" and thus loses sight of the aspect of creating these different levels by changing between different perspectives.

A common practice of differentiating between sitting and lying on the couch attempts to make obvious the distinction between using language and action and to support this distinction. Thus, whatever is discussed while sitting shall serve the organization issues, i.e., the setting of the frame. Whatever we are talking about when the patient is lying on the couch is understood in terms of the transference. Acting while sitting, however, is a well defined field only at first glance. It does not remain like that because those so-called "organizational issues" shall be included again in the analysis of transference on a meta-level. It is just because of these repeated changes and translations between the different levels that the translation from the affective experience to comprehension and insight works.

Translation, however, can lead also in another direction: in order not to lose contact to the affective levels of experience when changing to the level of self observation and of reflection we often use metaphors, stories, and symbolic expressions. These can be taken from the shared everyday language of patient and therapist and establish a connection to the collective unconscious, according to Jung. Alternatively, they can originate from the history mutually experienced during therapy. Here, metaphors can be invented and form a private language for two that can combine experience and insight just by referring to the shared mutual history. This level of "language for two" of the transference-countertransference interaction (finally) has to be left again and put into the context of the wider scope of the patient's own history.

In the papers and discussions at the Symposium we were confronted with another aspect of translation: the question of how to represent improvisations, scenes, or sequences of a therapy. This is the question of scientific therapy research in general. Here it deals with how music therapy can be researched, made comparable, and even measured. Raising the question in this way requires that you put yourself outside of what is happening in the therapy. The actual therapeutic medium of the music has to be left (as well). Here, too, the point is changing perspectives and, at the same time, changing the medium to language. In principle, the music of an improvisation can also be quoted or commented on by music itself, but finally the whole improvisation can only be made comparable and be evaluated by changing to a new level. This is primarily the level of language which describes by using words.

There is a further problem, especially when considering music therapy. This relates to the question of how music can be fixed as sounds fade away and cannot be produced in a short version to recall them. Can we recall them by playing the whole improvisation again or by listening to the whole tape? Or are there other ways?

This problem seems to be specific to music therapy research only at first glance. In verbal therapies we are also confronted with this question. Is it necessary, for example, to listen to a whole transcript of a therapy session or is it also possible to communicate the essence of a session by choosing a representative part of it? And the famous "first ten minutes" which are said to include everything that would follow during the session—are they sufficient to give a representative impression of the whole session? To what extent do different impressions result if there is only presented in the supervision what is thought to be most important or significant?

Before tape recording was introduced to therapies these questions were completely left to the mirroring processes of countertransference. This was partly because of the lack of exact means of reproducing sessions. But above all, psychoanalysts were convinced that what happens in therapy can be made comprehensible through the internal processes within the therapist and then be verbalized step by step by the analysis of the countertransference, thus increasingly approaching the level of secondary process.

By introducing raters in scientific research we can benefit from the internal information processing of countertransference reactions. Narrowing those reactions step by step by sticking to the theoretical presumptions is a way to translate between primary process material, such as the affective experience of the therapy session, and the more secondary process material, such as general theoretical statements.

In the study by Langenberg, Frommer, & Langenbach (1996) discussed in Monologue 6, this process of translation starts from the improvisation of the patient and therapist, leads to the affective countertransference reaction of the raters, then to the verbalization of these affects, then to figures, and last to graphic diagrams. The result is a gradual distancing from the original experience in the therapeutic session and leads to statements that are more and more general. In fact, this is the aim of scientific research.

On the other hand, by each step in translation the affective content of what has happened during the therapy sessions is gradually lost. Finally, the specific experience of the therapy session cannot be imagined and only general statements are retained.

In the study referred to above, during the research process there was a translation to graphic diagrams and thus a change to the level of pictures again. This could mean an increase in the intensity of affective representation, even though those diagrams are abstractions in a totally different manner. But in a more subtle sense we might prefer diagrams, not because of their digitalized, mathematical information, but because of their gestalt, which provides information on a symbolic level. Here we are in the field of metaphors again.

At the presentation of the research findings by Langenberg, Frommer, and Langenbach at the Symposium, the audience suggested that the raters should not make tables and diagrams at all. They preferred the raters to paint real pictures that could reproduce the affective content of the countertransference reaction and of the therapeutic situation in a more suitable way.

Even if this should diminish the content of the general statement for the individual therapeutic situation itself, patient and therapist could take advantage of the adding of a second non-verbal medium beneath music. This could also lead to more insight and enhance the therapeutic process.

Now we have to specify our question about the role of translation in the different therapies. It is about the direction and the number of the necessary steps. These depend on the aim in question. For scientific research aiming at general statements, more steps of translation towards the secondary process level are required than would be useful for supervision, for example. The latter should stay closer to the experience as the priority is the search for individual patterns in the interaction of the patient and the therapist and the transference-countertransference relation. Above all, for the patient-therapist interaction in the therapy process itself, we need an oscillating, changing, and translating between more primary process and more secondary process levels, thus using more metaphors and symbols or descriptive words providing information of a more general nature. Proceeding from the original experience during the therapeutic session: the more steps of translation, the more secondary process transformation, the bigger the increase in general evidence. On the other hand, if we stick to few steps in translation, we can better maintain the connection to the primary process affective experience of the therapy.

*   *   *

A man visits a group of polar researchers that has been on a research station for a long time separated from the rest of the world. In the evening they all meet and tell stories. The visitor realizes that, in turn, each of the men men says a number that makes the others burst into laughter. So he tries it, too: "Twenty-nine." Embarrassing silence. Being amazed, he asks and is told: "We tell jokes every evening. But we have heard them from each other so often that we only have to mention the number of the joke. Then we know." "And 'twenty-nine,' Why did nobody laugh?" "Well, it depends on how you tell a joke."

REFERENCES

Langenberg, M., Frommer, J. & Langenbach, M. (1996). Fusion and separation: Experiencing opposites in music, music therapy, and music therapy research. In M. Langenberg, K. Aigen & J. Frommer (Eds.), *Qualitative research in music therapy: Beginning dialogues*. Phoenixville, PA: Barcelona Publishers.

Qualitative Methods in Music Therapy Research: Epistemological Considerations

Michael Langenbach & Andreas Stratkötter

The use of qualitative research has gained momentum within psychotherapy research during the last two decades (Faller & Frommer, 1994). This is due both to researchers' and clinicians' increasing awareness of the limitations and shortcomings of comparative outcome research and a stronger interest in the therapeutic process.

This process cannot adequately be studied by experimental design and the testing of hypotheses under constant conditions. The most interesting variables in the therapeutic process are linked together by closely interrelated meaningful connections. Meaning, however, is something contextualized within the symbolic forms and cultures of human interactions. A process of description and analysis that proceeds inductively is more appropriate than experimental research in catching the meaning and symbols of human interactions and intrapsychic representations. The paradigm of constant conditions within the laboratory has to be replaced by a more idiographic, subject- and field-oriented approach which is provided by the means and concepts of qualitative research.

It is not a surprise that the qualitative movement has captured the interest of music therapy researchers as well. In music therapy, a symbolically transmitted social interaction takes place between individuals. To understand these interactions, a set of transformations based on hermeneutic and contextualizing interpretation is required by participants in the therapeutic interaction and by researchers looking at the therapeutic dyad.

Psychotherapy, in general, and music therapy, in particular, happen between two subjects who are empirical users of folk language. The usual step taken in research (both quantitative and qualitative) in psychotherapy is to transform the folk language into what is considered to be a more scientific or objective language. Qualitative methods, e.g., the grounded theory approach by Glaser and Strauss, emphasize the epistemological link between folk thinking and scientific thinking (Hildenbrand 1991). The process of transformation is, by necessity, theory-informed and led by the specific goals of an investigation (Langenbach, 1993). Compared to quantitative studies, the qualitative approach is more comprehensive and more adequate to the symbolic character of the material of music therapy sessions.

At the starting point of an increasing number of qualitative research programs in music therapy, there is a necessity to undertake an investigation of methodological and epistemological considerations. Henk Smeijsters (1996) tries to undertake this in his Monologue in the present text by attempting to link qualitative research to traditional parameters of good and valuable quantitative research.

We agree with Henk Smeijsters (1996) that it is a reasonable purpose to reflect upon (qualitative) research methods concerning their utilization in the field of music therapy. Of course, it is helpful to have a look at related scientific disciplines and to examine if sociology, psychology or other sciences may contribute certain methods or even methodologies to music therapy research. Qualitative single-case research surely promises to be a valuable concept when cautiously transferred to research into music therapy. Using qualitative approaches, similar transfers have be done by psychotherapy researchers in general, e.g., Rennie, Phillips & Quartaro, 1988.

Some points, however, in Smeijsters's paper on qualitative single-case research in music therapy deserve to be highlighted and put into perspective. First, Smeijsters's distinction between quantitative and qualitative research is a rather coarse one and may be misleading. Qualitative and quantitative research are not two completely different, mutually exclusive worlds, nor can quantitative research be seen as either the devil or a further development of qualitative research. Research into the processes of music therapy has to take into account that it is looking at a field which is artificial and man-made. The existing practice of music therapy is not nature. In such practice, conventions, social agreements, cultural phenomena, and subjective meaning are involved, whether explicitly or not. In this sense, practice and process are not theory-free but are also shaped by theory in the broad sense of culturally shared and subjective knowledge and opinions.

Second, a simple knowledge-truth-model in the sense of a representation theory which seems to shine through Smeijsters's paper cannot account for such a complex area of therapeutic interactions and strategies. Apart from the fact that contemporary epistemologists and critics of scientific method hold that there is no absolute truth which can be looked at more realistically by one or another method (Davidson, 1984; Rorty, 1991), it must be taken into account that by studying a field of human practice, theory and the participating observer with his/her network and concept of human relations are factors highly influential on the research process. An approach regarding human understanding as an artifact of socio-cultural discourses rather than a direct experience of ourselves is more appropriate when researching human matters (Gergen, 1985).

In our opinion, quantitative and qualitative research approaches do not follow two completely different kinds of research logic. Both methods afford transforming and interpreting processes (Faller, 1994). The distinction between calculative, quantitative use of theory, and descriptive, qualitative use of theory has to do with the methods of abstraction used. Quantitative research makes use of controlled, constant conditions, tries to eliminate uncontrollable variables as far as possible, and aims at statistical integration of the research results. Qualitative research is interested in the influences of conditions and variables and aims at a context-related integration of the research results. Description in qualitative research is not "more close to experience" as stated by Smeijsters (1996, p. 36). The concept of "experience" has to be qualified specifically for both qualitative and quantitative methods. Qualitative researchers are more interested in subjective experiences, whereas quantitative researchers try to establish experiences of general laws and rules, e.g., group-statistical connections.

Qualitative and quantitative approaches are both based in the assumptions of our shared social world. Researchers advocating for qualitative approaches have argued that qualitative research needs its own genuine set of criteria for judging the quality of research and have made reasonable proposals (Faltermaier, 1990; Mayring, 1990; Flick, 1987). In our opinion, a discourse about criteria for the quality of research in music therapy research is necessary. Spending much effort to prove different kinds of reliability and validity in single case approaches seems to be doing the second step before the first and, thus, perhaps choosing the wrong stairs.

REFERENCES

Davidson, D. (1984). On the very idea of a conceptual scheme. In D. Davidson (Ed.), *Inquiries into truth and interpretation*. Oxford: Clarendon Press.

Faller, H. (1994). Das Forschungsprogramm "Qualitative Psychotherapieforschung." Versuch einer Standortbestimmung. In H. Faller & J. Frommer (Eds.), *Qualitative Psychotherapieforschung: Grundlagen und Methoden*. Heidelberg: Asanger.

Faller, H. & Frommer, J. (1994). *Qualitative Psychotherapieforschung: Grundlagen und Methoden*. Heidelberg: Asanger.

Faltermaier, T. (1990). Verallgemeinerung und lebensweltliche Spezifitaet: Auf dem Weg zu Qualitaetskriterien fuer die qualitative Forschung. In G. Juettemann (Ed.), *Komparative Kasuistik*. Heidelberg: Asanger Verlag.

Flick, U. (1987). Methodenangemessene Guetekriterien in der qualitativ-interpretativen Forschung. In J. B. Bergold & U. Flick (Eds.) *Ein-sichten. Zugaenge zur Sicht des Subjekts mittels qualitativer Forschung*. Tuebingen: DGVT.

Gergen, K. J. (1985). The social constructionist movement in modern psychology. *American Psychologist, 40,* 266-275.

Hildenbrand, B. (1991). Vorwort. In A. Strauss (Ed.), *Grundlagen qualitativer Sozialforschung: Datenanalyse und Theoriebildung in der empirischen soziologischen Forschung*. Muenchen: Fink.

Langenbach, M. (1993). Conceptual analyses of psychiatric languages: Reductionism and integration of different discourses. *Current Opinion in Psychiatry, 6,* 698-703.

Mayring, P. (1990). *Einfuehrung in die qualitative Sozialforschung*. Muenchen: PVU.

Rennie, D. L., Phillips, J. R. & Quartaro, G. K. (1988). Grounded theory: A promising approach to conceptualization in psychology? *Canadian Psychology, 29,* 139-150.

Rorty, R. (1991). Is natural science a natural kind? In *Objectivity, relativism, and truth: Philosophical papers I.* Cambridge: Cambridge University Press.

Smeijsters, H. (1996). Qualitative single-case research in practice: a necessary, reliable, and valid alternative for music therapy research. In M. Langenberg, K. Aigen & J. Frommer (Eds.), *Qualitative research in music therapy: Beginning dialogues.* Phoenixville, PA: Barcelona Publishers.

A Psychoanalytic View of Music and Music Therapy Research

Gerhard Reister

As a naive lover of music who experiences musical sound, quite literally, in my body, it is quite difficult for me to enter into a scientific discourse about research in music therapy. This is also true for me as an empirical researcher in psychotherapy whose thinking is based on the nomological-deductive paradigm. As such, I intend to disclose causal regularities. I do not know much about qualitative research. Perhaps I have some proximity to its basic rules because I am, as a psychoanalyst, quite familiar with intentional-hermeneutic thinking.

In spite of all these confinements I should like to try to formulate some thoughts coming into my mind as an expectant participant of this inspiring Symposium and as a sympathetic reader of the papers presented.

To start with, I would like to say something about my personal view of music. This is my psychoanalytically informed understanding of what music provokes in listeners.

It seems that no one is able to escape the all encompassing effect of music so closely combined with emotions and emotional experience, i.e. inner-psychic processes which psychoanalysis aims to make understandable. There are two objective difficulties in this understanding:

First, whereas literary and scientific languages are enlisted into logical and discursive thinking even in its structure, the musical message is mediated without words and concepts (Kohut, 1955). Music reveals itself by presentative symbols (Langer, 1951; 1967) and has, in contrast to spoken language, the power to carry diverse contents at the same time. Thus, music is largely unapproachable (Haesler, 1991) for discursive language because of its prelinguistic and prelogical origins.

Second, music, especially without lyrics, is an "objectless art" (Sterba, 1946, p. 68), and eludes conception. Therefore, analyzing the forms and structures of music, while neglecting its content, would lead to an artificial dichotomizing into content-art and form-art, thus losing the vital music. As far as I know, even musicologists have not succeeded in formulating a theory of significant form defining the artistic form in tracing it back to content analysis.

Considering this, there is no reason for a kind of omnipotent fantasy that psychoanalytic discourse alone can explain the nature of music. Psychoanalysis, however, offers some deepening insights on this issue. One should notice that changes in psychoanalytical considerations on music parallel the development of psychoanalytic theory in general.

In the beginning, the psychoanalytical understanding of music was affected by libido theory. Music was considered to be a derivative of the id as the expression of originally instinctive wishes. It was to be perceived only indirectly because of sublimation processes and refinement by artistic and aesthetic means. In this view, musical pleasure derived from the listener's ability to perceive or sense the latent wishes in the musical structure and in the musical sound on a symbolic level. Bardas (1917/19) believes that music is speaking to the deep layers of the soul. Teller (1917/19) emphasizes in this context the "releasing effect upon displaced wishes" of sound (p. 13).

Musical sound also stimulates the development of fantasies in the listener. The early psychoanalytic theories distinguished between fantasies of omnipotence and imaginations in general. The former are, as Margolis (1954) states, to be found primarily in jazz music as "regressive narcissistic libido under the influence of the pleasure principle" (p. 286). Auto-erotic and narcissistic drives, however, are developmentally early forms of inner life. Thus, the emergence of such phenomena in adults is interpreted as a regressive process, i.e., a return to childlike modalities of psychic functions.

According to this theory, composing, playing and listening to music take place in regressive states with emotional experiences dominating logical and critical thinking.

Haesler (1982, 1991) rightly doubts that there is a general induction of regressive processes by music because its functions do not wear out in a direct access to unconsciousness. This line of interpretation has gradually gained momentum in the psychoanalytic literature about music. In particular, the structural model with its differentiation between id, ego and super-Ego, as well as the ego-psychological findings in the development of psychoanalytic theory allowed a more sophisticated consideration of musical expression and experience.

Menninger (1938) and Sterba (1939) thought that it was the function of all kinds of art to neutralize destructive tendencies and to organize the concepts of one's person and of the environment. Artistic activities would be a function of the ego, then. Music would be much more than an indirect expression of basal energies and latent wishes alone. Consciously experienced musical stimuli would be without any meaning or would ask too much of the listener if perceived by an ear not able to organize them.

Only Kohut and Levarie (1950) explicitly brought up formulations in this regard. The central assumption of their studies refers to the hypothesis, that the ego on the lowest level of development and of psychic functioning responds with fear to the musical sound which threatens to inundate the listener.

They suggest that the ego masters the musical stimuli by organizing and interpreting its structures which eventually leads to the enjoyment of music. They attribute a defensive force against endangering acoustical impressions to the ego.

In two brilliant papers, Kohut (1955; 1957) scrutinizes the inner psychic processing of music using the structural model of psychoanalysis. He demonstrates how music gives equal satisfaction to needs of the ego, superego and of the id:

1) Music is an emotional experience and thus allows for a cathartic dissolving of primitive impulses from the id;

2) Music can be understood as a play concerned with enjoyably organizing and structuring musical stimuli which is a function of the ego;

3) Music is an aesthetic experience using particular formal structures, to which one submits—it is thus an aspect of the superego with its norms and rules.

More recent developments in psychoanalytic metapsychology, such as narcissism theory or object relations theory, are not yet reflected in psychoanalytic literature about music. Nevertheless, the addictive use of music, for example, serves the defense and avoidance of a frustrating reality and stimulates the development of fantasies of a heavenly world of simple harmony. This could be called narcissistic and objectless.

What does all this mean for the psychoanalytic understanding of musical experience?

Freud (1914) laid the blame for his resistance to "being affected (by music) and not knowing why and what is affecting me" in his "rationalistic or maybe analytic aptitude" (p. 172). Thus, he is the prototype of the epicritical music receiver. This one directs his principal attention to the musical structures, e.g., motifs, melody, rhythm, etc., and tries to recognize these structures. Musical enjoyment then derives from (re-)perception and the ability of defining formal and aesthetical categories of music. Here, ego functions predominate against an excessive grasp or even attack of the music on proscribed or feared drive wishes, fantasies or emotions. Epicritical music listeners can develop an intensive love of the music of, for example, Johann Sebastian Bach, which, in works such as his fugues, is constructed quite mathematically. To follow this construction while listening may be an intellectual accomplishment. This kind of music reception allows for the fulfillment of superego needs.

If music is a vehicle for the expression of feelings, then instinctive drives should have an effect on the musical sound. Listeners open to this are experiencing a more intensive approach to those hidden impulses, wishes, and fantasies of the id depending on the depth of regression. They directly feel the "releasing effect of sound upon displaced wishes" (Teller 1917/19, p. 13), as in dreams or daydreams. This relaxing regression in the service of the ego—the protopathic music experience—can primarily be a sensual pleasure. It requires rational analysis which are not in the focus of the listener's interest because changes in the perception of reality would not be possible otherwise. According to Kris (1952), music, like other arts, displaces the boundaries of reality and replaces the everyday world by a world of illusion. The question is to what extent the resultant "aesthetic illusion" (Rauchfleisch 1986) can reach without this condition being experienced as intolerable. Probably "the controlling and directing functions of the id ought not be jeopardized" (Kris, 1952, p. 63).

The example of my patient Mr. K. may show this danger inherent in music. Suffering from a schizoid personality, he had severe problems in everyday life in being aware of his feelings and even greater difficulties in expressing them. With music, it was quite different: In the opera house especially he experienced ecstatic states with, in some cases, very impetuous emotional shocks. He then imagined fusing with the singers on stage and could in that way live his own impulses, mainly those of an aggressive nature. Several times after those experiences he suffered from states of derealization and depersonalization lasting for some hours.

One perhaps can find the fascination of music within this range between deep regression and rational analysis of musical structures.

I wonder whether or not music therapists and researchers would agree with these considerations. I suppose that in the Monologues of Carolyn Kenny (1996) and Dorit Amir (1996) there is something similar to my thoughts. Kenny is telling us something about abstract patterns which arise in music therapy more or less by themselves. However, she speaks about the necessity to build conceptual and theoretical structures to be able to understand musical experience. Does that not sound like proto-pathical and epicritical music experience? And does the cultural context so essentially implied not lead us to superego structures, to our habits of listening to music which we are familiar with, to our being embedded in a community of mutually shared cultural creeds providing security? The field of play may represent the space in which the ego is in enjoyable contact with the other, without words, only by the means of music.

The young patient of Dorit Amir gets out of her speechlessness by this process. She develops relation through the transitional object music and is then able to show something of her (aggressive) impulses.

Mechtild Langenberg, Jörg Frommer, and Michael Langenbach (1996) show such and similar effects in their Monologue in a very elaborated way. This paper clearly demonstrates that qualitative single case studies really dissect individual correlations beyond generalized correlational statistics, much like examining the process under a microscope. Thus, classification of inter-subjective correlations, interpretation of meaning, and the understanding of intrapsychic and interpersonal communication are all possible.

Kenneth Bruscia (1996) and Henk Smeijsters (1996) illustrate the methodological obstacles and pitfalls combined with this kind of qualitative research. Their Monologues, similar to Kenneth Aigen's (1996), go far beyond the boundaries of music therapy research. Bruscia's concept of authenticity pleases me personally. He demonstrates the importance of the researcher's personal interests in the results of his research activity. In that way he counters the belief in an abstract objective truth independent from man to which some natural scientists still profess belief.

Kenneth Aigen clearly demonstrates that qualitative research in music therapy must not be arbitrary and based upon the individual fantasies and biases of the researcher. Who could disagree with his comments about the importance of values?

Let me conclude by citing Sterba (1965): "The combination of and interaction between deepest regression and highly developed organization makes music a unique experience" (p. 111).

REFERENCES

Aigen, K. (1996). The role of values in qualitative music. In M. Langenberg, K. Aigen & J. Frommer (Eds.), *Qualitative research in music therapy: Beginning dialogues.* Phoenixville, PA: Barcelona Publishers.

Amir, D. (1992). *Awakening and expanding the self: Meaningful moments in the music therapy process as experienced and described by music therapists and music therapy clients.* Doctoral Dissertation, New York University. UMI Order # 9237730.

Amir, D. (1996). Experiencing music therapy: Meaningful moments in the music therapy experience. In M. Langenberg, K. Aigen & J. Frommer (Eds.), *Qualitative research in music therapy: Beginning dialogues.* Phoenixville, PA: Barcelona Publishers.

Bruscia, K. E. (1996). Authenticity issues in qualitative research. In M. Langenberg, K. Aigen & J. Frommer (Eds.), *Qualitative research in music therapy: Beginning dialogues.* Phoenixville, PA: Barcelona Publishers.

Bardas, W. (1917/19). Zur problematik der musik. *Imago, 5*, 364-371.

Freud, S. (1914b). *Der Moses des Michelangelo.* GW, Bd. X. Frankfurt/M.: Fischer.

Haesler, L. (1982). Sprachvertonung in Robert Schumann's liederzyklus "Dichterliebe" (1840). Ein beitrag zur psychoanalyse der musikalischen kreativitaet. *Psyche, 36*, 908-950.

Haesler, L. (1991). Zur psychoanalyse der musik und ihrer psychody namischen und historischen urspruenge. In F. Eickhoff & W. Loch (Hrsg.), *Jahrbuch der Psychoanalyse, 27,* 203-223.

Kenny, C. B. (1996). The story of the field of play. In M. Langenberg, K. Aigen & J. Frommer (Eds.), *Qualitative research in music therapy: Beginning dialogues.* Phoenixville, PA: Barcelona Publishers.

Kohut, H. (1955). Some psychological effects of music and their relation to music therapy. *Journal of Music Therapy, 4,* 17-20.

Kohut, H. (1957). Observations on the psychological functions of music. *Journal of the American Psychoanalytical Association, 5,* 389-407.

Kohut, H. & Levarie, S. (1950). On the enjoyment of listening to music. *Psychoanalical Quarterly, 19,* 64-87.

Kris, E. (1952). *Psychoanalytic explorations in art.* New York: International University Press.

Langenberg, M., Frommer, J. & Langenbach, M. (1996). Fusion and separation: Experiencing opposites in music, music therapy, and music therapy research. In M. Langenberg, K. Aigen & J. Frommer (Eds.), *Qualitative research in music therapy: Beginning dialogues.* Phoenixville, PA: Barcelona Publishers.

Langer, S. K. (1951). *Philosophy in a new key.* New York: Mentor Books.

Langer, S. K. (1967). *Mind: An essay on human feelings.* Baltimore, MD: John Hopkins Press.

Margolis, N. M. (1954). A theory on the psychology of jazz. *American Imago,* 11, 263-291.

Menninger, K. (1938). *Man against himself.* New York: Harcourt, Brace.

Rauchfleisch, U. (1986). *Mensch und musik: Versuch eines bruecken-schlages zwischen psychologie und musik.* Winterthur: Amadeus.

Smeijsters, H. (1996). Qualitative single-case research in practice: a necessary, reliable, and valid alternative for music therapy research. In M. Langenberg, K. Aigen & J. Frommer (Eds.), *Qualitative research in music therapy: Beginning dialogues.* Phoenixville, PA: Barcelona Publishers.

Sterba, R. (1939). Die problematik des musikalischen geschehens. *Imago*, 24, 428-433.

Sterba, R. (1946). Toward the problem of the musical process. *Psychoanalytical Review*, 33, 37-43.

Teller, F. (1917/19). Musikgenuß und phantasie. *Imago*, 5, 8-15.

Epilogue

Mechtild Langenberg
Jörg Frommer
Michael Langenbach
Kenneth Aigen

This book is being published in 1996, two years after an inspiring Symposium in Düsseldorf. The meeting itself and the process of compiling the various papers, editing them, and staying in contact over thousands of miles among numerous participants has revealed similarities, shared problems, and differences among the researchers involved. The similarities and tensions between different views have enriched our understanding of qualitative research in music therapy. We feel encouraged to continue this approach by enlisting a growing community of qualitative music therapy researchers who will form a vital multicultural group with different backgrounds as clinicians, artists and researchers.

Building Bridges Between Understandings was the title of David Aldridge's moderation of the final roundtable discussion at the Symposium. We feel that this is an appropriate title for the Symposium as a whole. Individuals met there for the first time who had read each other's work and who were struck by the similarities between them, even though they were developed in different parts of the world.

Main themes of discussion were highly varied, including the following: the importance of subjectivity and authenticity as attitudes of perception in a therapeutic setting and as instruments of understanding the research process; reflections about one's cultural identity as an important influential factor upon treatment, research, and the process of interacting at the Symposium; and, methodological considerations regarding the basis of qualitative research in music therapy. In the months following the Symposium, the dialogue continued, both on an internal level as the participants returned to their respective homes, and externally as the active and passive participants at the symposium continued their communications. The search for one's own identity became more prominent for certain researchers as a result of the cross cultural meetings at the symposium. Others emphasized that there should be more integration, resonance and translation of their experiences.

258 *Epilogue*

Throughout the Symposium and the dialogue process afterwards, the attempt was made to develop a culture of research meeting the high standards and guidelines typical of research in psychotherapy. Throughout this book, the high standard of research in music psychotherapy is apparent in the complexity of the methodological issues arising in the context of specific research problems. The change of paradigm embodied in this book—to one comprising single case studies, process research, and the use of qualitative methods to examine the interactions in treatment and the context of interpretations—serves to uncover the personal constructs of the researchers.

We feel that this book contains important original contributions which reveal that there are at least two vital methodological streams of thought in qualitative music therapy research, thus mirroring research trends in other disciplines such as psychology, sociology, and education. One complicating factor in determining into which group individual researchers fall is that the two positions are often not held in a pure form. Thus, an individual researcher or research team might have a perspective on data analysis and the role of the researcher's self, for example, that is characteristic of one group, while the use of narrative forms seems more typical of a contrasting group. Nevertheless, the following description can provide insight into some of the differences observed in this book.

In one perspective, researchers can set out their arguments *ad personam*, consider qualitative research as a search for authentic evidence, and maintain that they are more concerned with uncovering meaning rather than searching for objective truth. The other perspective is characterized by attempts to find and employ methodological analogies to quantitative research, while defining qualitative research as a rule-guided reconstruction of meaningful connections of material produced by research efforts.

The first type of methodological thought is based on the belief that traditional quantitative research—by virtue of its foundation in positivist and nomothetic tenets—fails to catch important aspects of subjectively and intersubjectively constituted reality. Researchers who hold this belief tend to utilize all realms of human experience as vehicles for data-gathering and analysis, including intellectual, non-verbal, affective, intuitive, and empathic modes. The starting points of such studies can be the mutually created meaningful moments existing within and between clients and therapists. Researchers of this kind acknowledge the cultural influences upon their research activity and products, such as the presence of individual and group values. They emphasize the importance of self-reflection, personal authenticity, and moral integrity as components of research methodology and have an expansive view of what constitutes an ethical concern in research, framing issues as a matter of ethics where other researchers would consider a particular concern a matter of research methodology without ethical implications.

Although these researchers make no claim to possessing a higher moral authority than quantitative researchers, some might conclude that this is implied by the way in which ethical implications are attributed to methodological choices. However, it is important to consider that an obligation to engage in a thorough pursuit of truth—considered either as a singular or a multifaceted phenomenon—is an essential ethical principle of all kinds of research and is, arguably, a criterion of research success. It is the sharing of this common search that mitigates against the ethical superiority of a particular research approach.

A danger in this type of research is that the freedom and flexibility in data analysis and interpretation afforded to the researcher is misused and becomes a license for the researcher to put forth personal speculation as the product of systematic research. This can occur when criteria for establishing the trustworthiness of findings are not engaged in with thoroughness and/or integrity. Ideally, the constructions and interpretations put forth in this type of research faithfully reconstruct the data provided by research participants. Whether or not these researchers are concerned with validity, per se, it is still essential in producing quality research that the conclusions are warranted by the original documents, including text, audio tapes and video tapes.

This type of research is often focused on finding embedded meaning in the surface presentations of patients, clients, therapists, and members of a research panel, much as a psychotherapist or psychoanalyst searches for latent meaning rather than what is directly manifest. What is considered the essence, theme or motif of a research participant's communications is inferred from an intensive and expansive interpretation of pieces of text which can be small in relation to the entire mass of data. When done well, this type of research can provide insight into internal processes in therapy and illuminate the meaning and significance of events.

Again, there is a danger, however, that the participant's communications are ignored or distorted because they conflict with those of the researcher. Then the participant's truth is minimized as the researcher assumes an authoritarian pose as the arbiter of truth, making far-reaching and unsupported interpretations from the surface of a text to an unconscious, core message. The rights of the individual research participant can be violated in this way.

In the second methodological view, qualitative research is seen as a variation of traditional research. This means that the standards for quality assessment of nomological research are still valid, albeit in a modified version. As with the first group, the researcher's observations of subjective experiences of patients comprise more than the personal opinions of the researcher. However, in the first group, idiosyncratic factors are not necessarily seen as distorting the research process if they are managed credibly; with the second group of researchers, an attempt is made to minimize the effect of any and all idiosyncratic factors.

Something common to both groups is the attempt to document the research process in detail, allowing the recipient of the study to detect conflicts and gaps in the chain of evidence between raw data and their interpretations and elaborations. This process is not dissimilar to the process of reading a detective story. Researchers in the second group extend this ideal out of a concern for replicability and tend to use research designs which allow for repeated analysis of the same data by other researchers. In methodological discussions much emphasis is placed on the fact that qualitative research does not employ quantification and statistical mean values in order to compare, prove, and generalize individual findings, instead employing more rhetorical and other narrative forms of presentation.

In both forms of qualitative research researchers value creating theories that are closely tied to research data, typically called grounded theory. Yet, as with all aspects of the research process, researchers in the first group give more latitude to, and pronounce a greater reliance upon, the researcher's self. This is also true in the activity of developing theory. Thus, while researchers in the first group tend to believe that seeking truly objective descriptions upon which to build theory is a misguided ideal, researchers in the second group put great weight on obtaining what they consider to be unequivocal, objective accounts of research subjects' opinions and attitudes. Qualitative researchers of both types make every effort to ascertain the subjective experiences of research participants and to systematically condense these accounts to render them in a clear and accessible fashion. Where the two approaches differ is in the degree of contribution the researcher can make to interpretations and theories arising from data. The first group sanctions a very active and interventive role on the part of the researcher, as long as it is implemented in a forthcoming manner; the second group tends to value the presentation of the information gleaned from a study with a minimal amount of contribution or interference from the researcher so that the final presentation is as faithful as is possible to the original data.

Again, if not done well, this second type of qualitative research can lead to studies where essential and underlying messages and meanings are obscured. Moreover, it is possible that incomplete analysis can lead to presentations which do not go far enough beyond the data and do not illuminate factors which are not already apparent in the texts comprising the data base. Last, it is possible that what emerges from these studies is kind of pseudo-reliability, mimicking the activity of quantitative researchers but ultimately relying on multiple subjective viewpoints which cannot, in principle, be raised to the level of the objective.

*   *   *

There are musical forms which are based on distinctive differences between two or more motifs, sections or characters, such as the sonata form, a compound binary form. These forms develop a process of tension resolution through the mutual exchange of ideas and mutual stimulation which usually flow into a conclusion of relaxed review. There is a sense of an achieved success, as the musical problems and tensions are resolved.

The differences between the two approaches in qualitative research are presented here in a somewhat coarse and exaggerated manner. There are, in reality, transitional motifs, developmental parts, and dialogues. The distinction between methodological understanding of qualitative research as evidence-oriented and as method-oriented may be used productively to answer concerns of how to ensure an understanding of holistic structures and hidden connections of meaning in an intersubjectively accessible way. In order to find answers to these questions the discussions among researchers with different approaches should continue.

Perhaps music therapy and music therapy research can learn from musical forms to use the potential of tensions between different motifs and characters for the benefit of the larger whole and for making progress toward better understanding our patients and ourselves and what we are doing when we conduct qualitative research.